Female Authority

FEMALE AUTHORITY

Empowering Women through Psychotherapy

POLLY YOUNG-EISENDRATH
FLORENCE L. WIEDEMANN

THE GUILFORD PRESS
New York   London

© 1987 The Guilford Press
A Division of Guilford Publications, Inc.
72 Spring Street, New York, N. Y. 10012

Printed in the United States of America

This book is printed on acid-free paper

Last digit is print number   9 8 7 6 5 4

Library of Congress Cataloging-in-Publication Data

Young-Eisendrath, Polly, 1947–
    Female authority

    Bibliography: p.
    Includes index.
    1. Women—Mental health.   2. Women—Psychology.
3. Power (Social sciences).   4. Psychoanalysis.
5. Psychotherapy.   I. Wiedemann, Florence L.
II. Title.
RC451.4.W6Y68   1987   155.6'33   86-27145
ISBN 0-89862-679-X
ISBN 0-89862-460-6 (paperback)

For   Jane Loevinger, my teacher
Frances Young, my mother
Amber, my daughter
Florence, my friend
   —*Polly Young-Eisendrath*

For my clients who taught me as we developed together, and for my friend and coauthor, Polly Young-Eisendrath, for whom I feel great admiration and love. And for all the women in my life who have given me their love, courage, wisdom, and inspiration.

   —*Florence L. Wiedemann*

ACKNOWLEDGMENTS

Many people must be thanked and acknowledged as having been part of this project. Foremost are the women clients with whom we have worked over the last 15 years. These women invented terms and contributed concepts which led to our discoveries and insights. Most notably, we thank the women whose material appears in the extended cases of Pandora and Psyche.

Bryn Mawr College generously provided Polly Young-Eisendrath with a faculty research award so that she could be freed from her teaching duties for one academic year in which the materials for this book were assembled and partly organized. She thanks the college for its support and specifically thanks Phillip Lichtenberg, Wendell Cox, and Mary Pat McPherson for their unique and vital inspirations and friendship in the process of writing this book.

Connie Sekaros, on the first round of editing, and Ernie Tremblay, on the second, did superb work in trimming off the bulk and making the text more readable. Ernie deserves special appreciation for his success in meeting deadlines and for his mindful editing of the lengthy case materials we assembled for Chapters 9, 10, and 11.

Two graduate students in Social Work and Social Research at Bryn Mawr, Lynne Mahan and Renee Balthrop, were outstanding assistants in keeping our scholarship tidy and accurate. Abstracting from books and journal articles, and meticulously checking our references, were the core of their efforts.

Natalie Everett and her Wayne Word Processing staff were efficient and accurate in all of the typing they did for us. We thank Natalie, Mary DeFrank, Debbie Smith, Judi Zwelling, and Pat Tyson, who typed the manuscript several times and gave us near-perfect copy at the end.

Paula Williams, personal secretary to Florence L. Wiedemann, was wholly competent and caring in every project she carried out. We thank her for her accurate typing, her diligent work on permissions, and her coaching of us when we were down.

Carl Jung, whose psychology of individuation is uniquely suited to understanding female development, is the archetypal Great Father in our background. His therapeutic discoveries in working with middle- and later-life people, and his astonishingly modern concepts of therapeutic influence, have too often been overlooked or misunderstood by American psychotherapists. We hope we have done justice to presenting a clear and accurate account of his complex understanding of symbolic development in human life. Jane Loevinger, Young-Eisendrath's major professor in graduate school, has had the greatest influence of any living psychological theorist on the overall conceptualization of this book. Her research and concepts of ego development provided us with a basic scheme for thinking about stages of animus development. Furthermore, her ego development scheme is part of the method of clinical assessment we use in our competence model. Her work on the psychology of women began with her investigations of Authoritarian Family Ideology over 30 years ago. She is an outstanding woman psychologist, a highly original thinker, and a careful scientist. We are especially grateful for her work.

We are grateful also to Demaris Wehr, a friend and professional colleague in feminist theology. She was an early collaborator on the manuscript. Although we eventually excluded (due to problems of space) her very intelligent critique of Jung's psychology, we are indebted to her for many of the ideas that spawned our revisions of Jung's psychology.

Pendle Hill Quaker Study Center was the setting in which we met to talk about this book during the early months of sharing ideas. The staff and students at Pendle Hill provided friendship, support, and silence in the long period in which most of this book was drafted during intensive writing retreats there.

Our family members have been more than generous and tolerant. They have been accepting, appropriately critical, and intelligent in their responses to this manuscript. Fred Wiedemann provided careful readings and suggestions. He is to be thanked especially for encouraging his wife toward an increasing acceptance of her female authority. She is most grateful for his encouragement during times when her confidence was failing.

Ed Epstein, husband of Polly Young-Eisendrath, has been an ever-ready sounding board and editor. Working in cotherapy with couples, presenting workshops and lectures together, and talking endlessly on car trips, he has provided stimulating occasions for discovery. As a partner, Ed combines the right ingredients for collaborative feminism:

humor, insistence, imagination, challenge, respect, and open-mindedness. Polly is grateful.

Polly's children, Amber, Colin, and Noah, have generously offered ideas, opinions, and argument. Amber was encouraging and inspiring, sometimes dubious, about the effects of feminism on her life. Colin wondered aloud how an 11-year-old boy could survive the embarrassment of telling his friends his mother had written a book with this title. Noah was patient and sympathetic in listening to the problems of manuscript preparation. All three children have been exceptionally patient in responding to their mother's edginess on writing days. Their love has always increased her courage.

Finally we thank the American Jungian community, especially the Inter-Regional Society of Jungian Analysts, who have made possible dialogues and debates on the topics at the core of this book. If we are to do justice to Jung's discoveries, surely we must make our own. In this way, we are not "Jungian," but we are our own authorities in contributing to a system of thought that was originally authored by Carl Jung.

Appreciation is expressed for permission to reprint excerpts from the following previously published material:

The psychological stages of feminine development by E. Neumann, *Spring*, 1959, 63–97. Reprinted by permission of Spring Publications, Inc.

The reproduction of mothering: Psychoanalysis and the sociology of gender by N. Chodorow. Reprinted by permission of University of California Press.

The self as agent by J. MacMurray. Reprinted by permission of Faber and Faber Publishers.

Life prints: New patterns of love and work for today's woman by G. Baruch, R. Barnett, and C. Rivers. Reprinted by permission of McGraw-Hill Book Company.

The collected works of C. G. Jung, trans. R. F. C. Hull, Bollingen Series 20, Vol. 16: *The practice of psychotherapy*. Copyright 1954, © 1966 by Princeton University Press; © renewed 1982 by Princeton University Press. Reprinted by permission.

Differentiation of gender identity by J. Money, *JSAS Catalog of Selected Documents in Psychology*, 1976, 6(4). Reprinted by permission.

In a different voice: Psychological theory and women's development by C. Gilligan. Published by Harvard University Press. Copyright © 1982 by Carol Gilligan. Reprinted by permission.

The madwoman in the attic: The woman writer and the nineteenth-century literary imagination by S. M. Gilbert and S. Gubar. Reprinted by permission of Yale University Press.

Work inhibitions in women: Clinical considerations by I. Stiver, *Stone Center Work in Progress Papers*, 1983, 82, 1–11. Reprinted by permission of Stone Center for Developmental Services and Studies, Wellesley College.

Collected papers on schizophrenia and related subjects by H. F. Searles. Reprinted by permission of International Universities Press, Inc.

Needed concepts in the study of gender identity by C. W. Sherif, *Psychology of Women Quarterly*, 1982, *6*, 378–388. Reprinted by permission of Human Sciences Press, Inc.

Collected papers, Vol. 3, by Sigmund Freud, authorized translation by Alix and James Strachey. Published by Basic Books, Inc., by arrangement with The Hogarth Press Ltd. and The Institute of Psycho-Analysis, London. Reprinted by permission.

The gods of the Greeks by C. Kerenyi. Copyright © 1979 by Thames and Hudson Ltd. Reprinted by permission.

Inventing motherhood: The consequences of an ideal by A. Dally. Reprinted by permission of Schocken Books Inc.

Myths of the Greeks and Romans by Michael Grant. Reprinted by permission of Weidenfeld (Publishers) Limited.

Language and insight by Roy Schafer. Reprinted by permission of Yale University Press.

"Diving into the wreck" and "The mirror in which two are seen as one" by Adrienne Rich. Copyright © 1984 by Adrienne Rich. Copyright © 1975, 1978 by W. W. Norton & Company, Inc. Copyright © 1981 by Adrienne Rich. Published in *The fact of a doorframe, Poems selected and new, 1950–1984* by W. W. Norton & Company, Inc. Reprinted by permission of the author and W. W. Norton & Company, Inc.

PREFACE

The desire to write this book arose from distress. As psychotherapists working with women clients, we were repeatedly confronted with women's lack of belief in themselves, lack of independent financial resources, lost opportunities for education and employment, despair about relationships with men and children, and, above all, insistent self-blame. In consequence, we found ourselves frequently wondering whether their feelings of helplessness were more authentic than our hope of helping.

Our years of training as psychologists and Jungian analysts had supposedly equipped us with theories and methods for understanding and helping. We came to realize, however, that we could no longer use only the tools and cognitive maps which were most familiar to us. Diagnosing psychopathology, applying standards for mental health and norms for gender and personal identity had inexorably led us to see our clients in terms of *deficits*. Thus, when we evaluated and interpreted the lives of these women from the traditional perspectives of psychodynamics and psychopathology, we unintentionally reinforced their internalized inferiority.

Although we might have responded to this insight in any number of ways, we focused on two issues which seemed critical to the problem. The first is a woman's relationship to her own authority, as it emerges in the context of her life experiences in a patriarchal society. In other words, how does a woman claim the validity of her own truth, beauty, and goodness as originating in her own experience? The second is the need to build a "competence assessment" model based on the concept of personal authority which can be used in general decision making for psychotherapeutic treatment. We have aimed to provide a model for systematic evaluation of strengths in the context of vulnerabilities and stress. Rather than assessing our clients primarily in terms of deficits (i.e., what is wrong with them), we look for what is adaptive and effective. Our goal is to extend our clients' strengths and expand these into new attitudes and activities, in the hope of empowering clients to deal with emergent challenges of meaning, motivation, and empathy in their everyday lives.

In this book we draw heavily on our own clinical practices in illustrating our efforts to help women assume their own authority. Although we have treated hundreds of women using this perspective, we have revealed as little as possible about the actual identities of the women we have seen. In other words, we have drawn on only a relatively small number of cases (about 25 from our combined practices) for specific details, and have combined many of these cases to make amalgams of actual women. In some instances, however, we have revealed specific and personal details about individual women's lives. Both out of respect for confidentiality and with the knowlege that exposure would be threatening to our current and past clients in therapy, we tread a fine line between giving actual observations and constructing illustrations from our experiences. Writing this book has reemphasized for us how problematic it is to use clinical material in a public forum. Whether the material is disguised, current or old, the intrusion into the private nature of psychotherapy is offensive. In this light, we have chosen actual details from cases where it seemed we could do the least harm. Naturally, the effort to conceal and obscure details has made the empirical nature of our observations difficult to represent. Had we been working on research *per se*, we might have felt more satisfied with our ability to give the exact details of individual cases. Our readers should know, however, that all dream texts and the two extended cases presented in Chapters 9, 10, and 11 are straightforward empirical representations, using the exact words of clients and the recorded materials from sessions. Other references to case materials, in terms of individual assessments and personal data (e.g., ages), have been presented in a way which protects personal identity while exposing essential clinical elements.

We hope that this book will liberate therapists to think about women (and perhaps men) clients in a new way. Assessment for treatment decisions and interventions using psychotherapy should be based on a nondeficit cooperative understanding with clients, an understanding which can be conveyed in ordinary language. In order to assist women in therapeutic treatment, we had to revise our assumptions about what women contribute to culture in all of the arenas in which they are involved. Understanding ourselves (as women) to be agents of our culture and our own lives renews our connection to symbolic meaning systems and cultural resources that will provide the foundation for feminist epistemologies. We hope that we have assembled our material in a way that is useful to psychotherapists and to women in general.

CONTENTS

1

Introduction

Personal authority is the ability to validate one's own thoughts and actions as good and true. It develops gradually as others recognize and communicate the value of one's ideas and contributions, both for the family and for the larger social group. Our society designates authority symbolically by conferring decision-making influence, social status, and power over material resources. These are typically not associated with women or women's work.

In the family as well as the professions, men have the advantage of greater managerial influence and control over material resources. Moreover, at the level of gender identity, males are socialized to feel and to behave authoritatively, while women form "identity relationships" with them in order to validate their own personal authority. In such relationships—whether with father, brother, husband, supervisor, son, or teacher—a woman maintains her self-esteem and personal worth primarily through male reflections.[1] The results are problematic for both women and men. Such relationships are often infused with the woman's anxiety and low self-esteem. In her desire to witness her own authority, validity, or goodness in male reflections, a woman may relate to a boy or man as an aspect of her identity rather than as a person in his own right.

Troubling as it is, when females identify with their own gender, they part from a sense of personal authority. In our society, we are constantly and everywhere subjected to the tacit assumption that males are superior, especially the normative white males often called "middle class." Implicitly and explicitly, male norms have become our social standards for health, mental health, leadership, relationships, and per-

1. Our uses of verb and noun forms of "reflect" and "reflection" often allude to a psychological meaning: the internalizing of a personal image, likeness, or attitude from what others give back, communicate, or imply about oneself.

1

sonal autonomy. Whether or not we as individuals accept these standards, we live in a society that organizes itself collectively according to them, and we are all influenced by them. Studies of Americans' expectations of "ideal" women and men, conducted by Broverman, Broverman, Clarkson, Rosenkrantz, and Vogel (1970) and Broverman, Vogel, Broverman, Clarkson, and Rosenkrantz (1972), are often cited as empirical evidence of the collective prejudices we share about gender differences. These studies showed that many Americans expected men to be stronger, more objective, more competent, and more independent than women—results that seem self-evident in our daily experiences.

Additionally, women were expected to be weaker, less competent, and more emotionally expressive and subjective than men. Ideals for adult female behavior included more dependence and less competence than those for a "healthy adult, sex unspecified." This revealing finding clearly shows how women are locked into a double bind in terms of their gender: If they behave as healthy adults, they are considered unwomanly, but if they behave as ideal women, they will be considered childlike or inferior.

As they are socialized into female gender identity, American girls and women are forced to develop a negative self-concept. The assumption of female inferiority (the "less than" characteristics) may be either revealed or hidden in an individual's adaptation, but it will somehow be central to her self-concept. All women in our society arrive at adulthood with significant feelings of inadequacy. These personal states of internalized inferiority are not simply occasional or transitory identity aspects. They are pervasive, inescapable ideas about one's inadequacy as a person. Typically, they are preoccupations with an inability to experience truth, beauty, or goodness in oneself and/or one's actions. Negative evaluations of body, attractiveness, intelligence, independence, competence, or nurturing are examples of the common experiences of a woman who feels herself inferior.

Gender categories, which sort people into different groups that carry symbolic meaning about personal ability and roles, exist in all known societies. These categories are mutually exclusive; that is, a person can be a member of only one category. Both male and female gender categories depict abilities, attitudes, and roles that are essentially human. Yet a person is permitted to identify with only one. Therefore, certain aspects of human identity are excluded from everyone's self-concept as belonging to the opposite gender.

We agree with Lipman-Blumen's (1984) argument that gender differences in our society provide the blueprint for most other power differences. Oppression of racial minorities, decision-making hierarchies in families and nations, and dominance of certain ethnic groups over others are only a few examples of social dominance modeled on beliefs about inherent differences in individuals' ability to will and direct their own lives.

Our society strongly supports the "blues and pinks" of gender identity even in infancy. From birth onward, the category of gender membership for most infants is clear. Personal actions, appearances, and abilities are marked by gender meanings. There is no other category of human difference that occurs so early and is carried so persistently throughout a person's lifetime.

PSYCHOLOGICAL REASONING ABOUT WOMEN: THE DEFICIT MODEL

Many of us who are human service providers, in psychology, social work, psychiatry, and education, unintentionally reinforce low self-esteem in girls and women. When we assess, evaluate, or treat a female as though her internalized inferiority is a fact or a personal fault, we increase feelings of powerlessness in her. The knowledge that women have acquired about themselves through psychology and sociology has, unfortunately, tended to reinforce negative self-concepts. Women are described as fearing success, lacking assertiveness and being emotionally immature and morally inferior.

Many women these days openly fight feelings of inferiority and inadequacy. Instead, they identify with strength, competence, and capability. Unfortunately, they have not escaped the double bind of gender identity because they are frequently seen and described (by both others and themselves) as compensating or too masculine. Socially, such a woman experiences an intense double bind concerning her insistent, forceful behavior and often reports hidden fears of inadequacy. She is likely to be perceived as problematic and distressing in environments of male authority. If a human service professional describes her as too controlling, demanding, rigid, and aggressive, these characteristics will become readily familiar to her, and she will easily label them as "problems" in her identity.

On the other hand, women who have accepted the traditional meanings of female gender as normative, and thus seem passive or submissive, face a different kind of double bind. They are perceived as adequately feminine and flexible, but are easily regarded as childlike and too dependent, especially by mental health professionals. Many syndromes of mental "disorders" are typified by exaggerated feminine characteristics: depression, hysteria, phobia, dependent personality, anorexia, bulimia, and certain aspects of psychotic behavior (e.g., borderline enactments of intense emotionality). Feminine-identified women who seek help at public mental health clinics, hospitals, and private services risk being labeled into categories of mental illness that suggest they are defective because they are excessively feminine.

Much current psychological reasoning about women is founded on androcentric thinking. Androcentrism, or seeing the world from the male perspective, results in mistaken assumptions and misleading questions about women. When we make assumptions about women based on men's experience of themselves or their relationships with women, we are reasoning androcentrically. Making inferences about women based on essentially male standards results in evaluating women through the wrong categories, usually in terms of how they are deficient or lacking in a quality or attitude that men value. For example, evaluating women by male standards for autonomy can result in labeling our entire sex as overly dependent or insecure when we are simply quite well connected to basic human needs for interpersonal contact.

Androcentric thinking is similar to a general style of logic, typical of many mental health professionals, which we call "deficit thinking." Deficit thinking directs our attention toward what is absent, deficient, or wrong in a person or situation. When a psychotherapist approaches a client to see "what's wrong," the therapist is engaging in deficit thinking. This kind of framework emphasizes weakness or problematic elements and de-emphasizes—or even ignores—strengths, and leads finally to the medical model of illness or distress.

NO BLAME: BEYOND THE DEFICIT MODELS

Inherent to the medical model is the implication that a person has been victimized by an external force (e.g., by bacteria or deprivations in parenting). Medical diagnosis (from symptom description to causal hypotheses) is especially counterproductive as an assumptive framework for treating women through psychotherapy. Women already feel victimized and rendered helpless in a variety of ways which interfere with making competent responses to their stresses and vulnerabilities. Additionally, they are socialized to look to the external environment, especially powerful males, to provide the means to life satisfactions. The illness model often reinforces the sense of defeat a woman experiences in trying to master the circumstances of her life. Locating the cause of a woman's distress primarily in terms of an external force (e.g., genetic inheritance of a mood disturbance) may actually contribute to her problems, especially her feelings of inadequacy.

Second, the interpretation of affective and cognitive difficulties in terms of illness ignores, or de-emphasizes, the current interactive social influences with which the woman is dealing in both her personal life and the larger culture. Human relatedness is the primary ground of both successes and problems in human living; relatedness also seems to be the central curative factor in all forms of therapeutic influence. Without a full consideration of relatedness, in both its social and symbolic forms, a therapist easily can feel overwhelmed and defeated in desiring to help a woman client, and may even be inclined to "blame the victim" by insisting on her resistance or her illness as a barrier to change.

The symptom approach to assessing problems in living delineates an understanding of personal life which is unfortunately syntonic with the framework many women bring with them into therapy. Clients come to therapy with elaborate rationales for what is wrong in their lives. They often make use of complex reasoning in order to identify faults or flaws within themselves or their parents which have led to current distressing effects. Moreover, clients have already rehearsed these blameful explanations to family and friends, and perhaps to other professionals as well. If blame and deficit thinking were useful motivations for change, then change would have occurred without therapy.

Besides the sense of hopelessness engendered by the illness model of psychopathology, and the accompanying blame orientation to life in general that it reinforces, many other assumptions of the model are erroneous. The concept of disease, with circumscribed symptoms, does not fit the three major foci of concerns presented by psychotherapy clients: (1) consensus about "reality" and other questions of *meaning*, expressed sometimes as distortions of perception and cognition; (2) problems of *empathy*, manifested by feelings of being misunderstood, rejected, or engulfed by other people; and (3) problems of *motivation*, manifested as despair, ennui, low self-esteem, and experiences of being worthless and useless to others.

Unfortunately, when a psychiatric label such as "borderline personality disorder" is affixed to a person, one tends to feel that something "scientific" has been done. We can easily believe that we have objectively isolated an ailment we can treat, when in fact we have done nothing more than reinforce a questionable system of nomenclature. Clearly, psychotherapists need a common language for assessment, treatment, and research. There is no justifiable rationale for using the language of psychopathology based on the medical model of disease. Not only is this language rooted in assumptions which mislead and overwhelm us in our efforts to enhance meaning, empathy, and motivation, but also, the scientific beliefs that reside in our use of the medical approach may blind us to our imprecisions.

Psychiatric diagnoses are not very precise or reliable. Even with the best possible descriptive categories of symptoms (e.g., some of the well-researched categories of the third edition of the *Diagnostic and Statistical Manual of Mental Disorders*; American Psychiatric Association, 1980), the labeling of disturbances is a matter of interpersonal consensus among practitioners. For most classifications of psychopathology there is considerable leeway for disagreement and, especially in the early stages of a "disorder," much room for error in judgment. All the same, practitioners often use the labels dogmatically. Clients come to us resigned to accept a lifelong disability called "depression," "agoraphobia," or "excessive dependency" much in the same way a person would be resigned to living with a chronic illness like diabetes. Whether or not they understand what the labels mean, the clients judge from the self-assured seriousness of the diagnostician that a scientific pronouncement has been made about the cause of their distress.

Treatment by psychotropic drugs,[2] which limit consciousness and activity, often follows diagnostic labeling and implies to the client that she can only be sustained by medication. The client may understandably mistake the medication for treatment of an underlying condition of illness, as an antibiotic would be used to treat a bacterial infection, but a more accurate medical analogy would be treatment of a cold with aspirin because the cold is not cured by the drug. Most of us know that aspirin masks symptoms of physical stress in such a way that it can be harmful to us if we ignore the underlying condition, but because we are all prone to believe in the miracles of science, clients readily suppose that drugs replace psychotherapy and improve their condition. In fact, the neurological and psychological effects of most psychotropic medications are not well understood, yet doctors who are not psychotherapists or even psychiatrists often prescribe these drugs without sufficient explanation. The medications are used to manage symptoms and reduce anxiety. They do not produce changes in interpersonal relationships but only reduce some of the emotional stress. Medications may help the client feel better, and thus have more resources available, but they can also lead to a dependency on doctors which replaces the vitality of human feeling and real contact with other people.

Finally, the medical routine of examining, diagnosing, and treating is simply not relevant to psychotherapy. Both our method of treatment and the difficulties we treat are interpersonal. We are not treating an illness or its symptoms; we are assisting people in developing new attitudes and meaningful perspectives on themselves so that they can become more useful and involved.

Our premise of nondeficit thinking about clients and its expansion into a system of evaluation are presented in Chapters 3 and 4 as we have come to use them to oppose self-blaming and other-blaming in psychotherapy. As we articulate and study the competences, skills,

---

2. Evidence, now well documented, indicates that women receive over 70% of prescribed psychotropic medications, including tranquilizers, sedatives, stimulants, and antidepressants (Hare-Mustin, 1983, p. 595).

adaptations, and talents of our clients, we slowly devise a system of primary prevention of psychological distress by understanding how people successfully meet the challenges of their lives. This is a distinctly different project from psychopathology, a record of human failings to meet the norms of a particular culture in its standards for success. If therapists use primarily a psychopathological approach to female clients' distress, both therapists and clients will constantly be immersed in negative images of clients as full of defects and losses which need to be fixed—in life contexts that seem to lack the necessary resources.

Psychotherapy, whether analytical or behavioral, depends on establishing a foundation of trust between therapist and client. From research on effectiveness of psychotherapy treatment, we have delineated several elements of interpersonal influence which mark the therapeutic relationship as effectively influential in assisting people to change. Psychotherapy involves at least four "nonspecific" factors of relationship. First, and foremost, an adequate *rapport* must be formed and managed between client and therapist. Rapport involves empathy and the power of one person to influence another through beliefs or emotional force. In psychoanalysis and psychoanalytic forms of therapy, the rapport is called the *transference* or *working alliance*. In family therapy, it is typically called *joining*. In behavioral and active therapies, the rapport is referred to as a *contract for treatment*. The other three nonspecific factors all contribute to the element of rapport and are common to all forms of therapy. The first is usually called the *placebo effect*. This is a client's belief that the treatment will work or will help. (A term from ordinary language for this factor is *hope*.) The second nonspecific factor of therapeutic influence is *suggestion*. Suggestion involves the authority that the client believes to be embodied in the therapist so that the therapist's direct advice, guidance, ideas, etc., seem powerful. The final nonspecific factor is *social ritual*, sometimes called the *therapeutic frame* or *group dynamics*. Social ritual of time, place, defined activities, and fee gives a circumscribed, agreed-upon social meaning to the meeting of therapist and client. This ritual, like a religious ritual, carries larger cultural meaning in terms of the curative effects of psychotherapy.

The relational or nonspecific factors of psychotherapy are not the only curative factors operating, but they are essential and important for both client and therapist.

If the disease model and deficit thinking are misleading orientations current among psychotherapists, what can be done to shift our approach in understanding and treating women? This book is our attempt to devise a systematic and comprehensive model of assessment for female clients, a model which links directly to decision making about treatment and incorporates a psychosocial understanding of the effects of internalized inferiority. We integrate a psychology of symbolic meaning, Carl Jung's psychology (for references, see next chapter), with a therapeutic orientation of egalitarian relationship (feminist therapy) in order to increase the possibility of enhancing competence and authority in women clients. We include other approaches which are consonant with our aims. Loevinger's (1976) ego development scheme is incorporated in our assessment process, and we make use of ideas from social psychology, object relations theory, and Piaget's cognitive psychology. Our central desire has been to devise a model which responds to women's conflicts in living in a patriarchy as they attempt to bring about change in themselves and their society.

We recognize that our model and our analyses are culture bound and may not be broadly applicable for understanding clients who are very different from the women we have treated in public and private agencies, and in independent practice. With that caveat in mind, we hope that we have something to say to all Americans who have been stereotyped as being inferior or deficient according to the white androcentric norms. A central theme in all the work we have done with women has been the fear of personal insignificance, which becomes associated with feelings and acts of depression, envy, jealousy, hatred, and aggression. Many adults in our society share in this distressing fear.

FEMALE AUTHORITY: OUR PERSPECTIVE ON WOMEN

The ability of a woman to validate her own convictions of truth, beauty, and goodness in regard to her self-concept and self-interest is what we call *female authority*. Body image, self-confidence, personal agency, social functioning, occupational functioning, sexual pleasure, and subjective self-assessment are all related to female authority.

We assume that all women who have reached adulthood in patriarchal society will evaluate themselves, even their strengths at times, from a deficit orientation. This perspective has been imposed through socialization, is constantly reinforced in everyday living, and must be compensated by understanding the meaning of female gender.

With this as background, we propose a model of female development which conceives of identity as evolving through a tandem relationship of self and other. Women, through their gender identity and social roles, are openly dependent on significant others for reflections of themselves. Through this identity in relationship, girls and women develop particular strengths and skills that permit them to understand and manipulate interpersonal cultural resources. For example, many women develop the ability to relate in nonrational modes of gestural, implied, and emotional expressions—and to infer interpersonal meaning from a wide range of signals often ignored by men. This is a skill which has been pejoratively labeled as "feminine intuition."

Another strength specific to female socialization is the power of emotional expressiveness. We will later take up the more complex issue of analyzing female power as experienced through emotional displays within the family. For the time being we would like to note that vital and poetic expression of feeling is an indicator of advanced female development. Open expressions of differentiated feelings have assisted women in understanding emotional dependence as essential to human life.

Finally, female development typically includes a concern for personal beauty, an aesthetic orientation to everyday life, which may be trivialized by commercial pandering of cosmetics manufacturers. When a woman has consciously integrated the power of her appearance as an aspect of her authentic identity, she has under her control a wide range of choices about how to express herself. This strength of female development has become so constrained by forced competition among women that most women find the topic of their appearance somehow belittling to their personal authority. Still, appearance is a central motif in female development and one which silently accompanies the relationship of mother to daughter over the life span.

As we mentioned earlier, we rely on several theoretical frameworks for characterizing our model of female development. From Loevinger's (1976) work on ego development, we assess the cognitive, interpersonal, and moral functioning of our clients' conscious female identity. Loevinger has delineated nine stages, summarized in Chapter 4, which can be used to understand the assumptions a woman makes about herself in relation to others, to ideals, and to society. From Carl Jung (1959), we have taken the concept of *animus*. We define animus as the excluded masculine aspects of a woman's conscious female self. We have used Jung's idea of animus and some of his psychology of individuation to understand the excluded masculine complex of authority and competence in a woman's personality. Women who grow up and are socialized in a patriarchal culture are forced to exclude authority from their self-concepts. They must retrieve it from experiences in the masculine world of culture and then convert these experiences to confidence in themselves. Because mothers are the primary and initial authorities in everyone's life, we assume that most girls and women once felt their own female authority, but lost it in the process of socialization and gender identity formation. In Chapters 2 and 3, we attempt to show why we must change our fundamental concepts for female personality (in our current culture of established therapeutic practice) and how we have come to understand it differently, in terms of female experience. As Chapter 3 shows, we have revised Jung's ideas substantially, but with an overall congruence with his basic assumptions. The Jungian assumption of personality as a dialectic of competing realities is persuasive as an adequate framework for female personality. A woman's ongoing sense of personal coherence and continuity (being) is a project of balancing and holding together opposite and competing self-references, both in the moment and over time. To experience herself as an independent decision maker (in childrearing and breadwinning, for example), she must emphasize certain aspects of her identity which may be in contrast to equally prominent ideals of yielding receptivity (as a wife or girlfriend, for example). To understand and articulate the basic conflicts in female identity between consciously claimed gender (as female) and unconsciously excluded animus (as the authority of the male "other") has been our central study in this book. Chapters 5 through 11 are mainly concerned with setting out our system for doing this and showing how we have come to use it in psychotherapy with adult women.

Our model for female development is essentially a conflict model. We assume that a women's identity is a conflicted self-system of competing roles, attitudes, and self-assessments. Inherent in her gender identity is a double-bind conflict about female authority, as we have already explained. Inherent in her traditional femininity are many conflicts about her relationship with her mother in terms of her mother's responses to her own internalized inferiority.

Underlying our model for female development is a central assumption that a woman must be successfully regarded by some significant men in her life in order to integrate the conflicting aspects of her identity. In her relations with significant males, she is initially forced (by norms of our society) to evaluate her own worth through patriarchal reflections. If her relationships with father, uncles, teachers, brothers, lovers, sons, and husbands produce primarily negative and abusive self-reflections, she will not be able to fully actualize her personal authority. Such authority, generated through a woman's authentic experience of herself, rather than through distorted and projected desires, must be lost and then retrieved in order to be integrated in a society of father rule.

Among adult women, the stages of ego and animus development which we present are best understood as typologies of difference. Some women continue developing through later stages and others do not. In adult life, different types of women are represented by different preoccupations, attitudes toward self and other, cognitive functioning, and the like. In the next chapters we present these models in detail.

The ability to validate one's own convictions is a dialectical process of relativism, responding differently in a variety of situations. We prefer the ideal of female authority to that of ego autonomy because the latter emphasizes independent individuality across a variety of situations. As an autonomous person, one imposes one's will and values on others. As an authoritative person, one responds flexibly to a variety of different desires and needs from self and others. The interactive process of a woman consciously in dialogue with both her interpersonal and her intrapsychic environments is our aim. Rather than maintaining a consistent set of self-attributes which she imposes on all situations, she strives for an ability to be both empathic and decisive in her responses to each new environment while she maintains a commitment to her own values.

Female authority is an achievement of adulthood that follows from projections of authority onto men and male institutions. Engendering female authority in a male-dominated society entails legitimatizing conflicting needs and desires, especially those concerned with approval and self-determination. Given her socialization, a female initially projects her self-validation onto men (because they possess the symbolic authority and hold the decision-making positions in our culture) and then retrieves it at some cost to her own personality. (She must come to terms with her own resistance and aggression.) The retrieval of female authority involves a renewed appreciation of female socialization, including the validation of her own perceptions and ideals as worthy although perhaps different from her male counterparts. Achieving a relatively coherent sense of self and a unified experience of one's own needs and values entails constant striving for women living in patriarchal society. In essence, the experience of a relatively coherent female self is an ongoing project of consciousness building that encompasses a woman's personal history and the history of female identity in her society.

Our ideals of optimal development in adulthood include both personal authority and androgyny. We believe that androgyny comes relatively late, if at all, in the process of female development. It is only after a woman has penetrated the meanings of both personal and cultural forms of female identity that she is ready for something like an authentic androgyny. Androgyny is not simply taking on male roles and attitudes. Rather it is the ability to be essentially human, and to choose for oneself the most authentic masculine or feminine gender modes, depending on the current environment. In order to sustain oneself and understand the opposing values and reference systems involved in androgyny, a woman must have a deep respect for, and trust of, the knowledge derived from conflict.

2

Conflict as Identity: Why a Woman Can't Be More Like a Man

Much deficit thinking about women has developed from the relatively simple idea that women want what men have because it is intrinsically better. Assumptions that males are superior have led us directly to hypothesize that women covet male attributes and even male biology: greater physical strength, greater financial resources, and the penis. Women's desires and needs are thus conceptualized, not as actual desires for sovereignty over their own lives, but as compensatory desires in reaction to men. Deficit thinking about the emotional power of women—labeled manipulative or overly controlling—often assumes that women are primarily reacting to what is missing in themselves rather than striving for their own coherence and validity.

The combined effects of deficit thinking and white male androcentrism have resulted in some seriously misleading ideas about female development. In approaching women from the point of view of male standards, we unintentionally obscure both the conflicts inherent in all women's identities as adults, and the strengths they need to work through these conflicts.

CONFLICTS IN THE FEMALE SELF-SYSTEM

Psychological reasoning about female identity still carries remnants of the now outdated position that "biology is destiny." Some contemporary authors (e.g., Stevens, 1982) continue to argue that female gender identity is closely bound to biological and hormonal dictates, which prepare a woman for her inherent role as nurturer. Similarly, these dictates (such as hormonal effects on status of mind) limit her functioning in other ways so that she is less likely to be a true carrier of culture.

Most psychologists and sociologists embrace an interactive model of sociobiological influences on gender identity, even if they do not carry out fully the assumptions of their position. We take a firm position that the ambiguity of biological and social factors influencing gender will never be clarified because contrasting the two presents a false opposition, a mistaken orientation toward the idea of gender. Gender is a sociobiological condition of symbolic meaning within a culture or society. Gender is not a set of sexual characteristics deriving from the structure of the human body. These characteristics are, in fact, aspects of gender symbolization. The penis stands for certain meanings within a culture, such as strength or reason. However, strength and reason do not derive from having a penis. Both biological and social factors are necessary for developing gender categories; they are interactive and evolving within the function of culture, the ways in which a culture shapes its individuals for particular roles.

In terms of the process of individual gender differentiation, the model here is also one of interaction. Certain biological conditions typically set the boundaries for gender attributions, and then sociocultural conditions influence the individual. Money (1976) provides a helpful analogy between gender differentiation and the acquisition of language:

> You can draw on this analogy of native language; you have to have certain dispositions in the brain pathways, but how you actually utilize those dispositions is going to be entirely dependent on social exposure, interaction, and experience. (p. 17)

Based on their research with babies whose gender was reassigned postnatally due to structural abnormalities, Money and Ehrhardt (1972) concluded that the major part of individual gender identity is "left by nature" to be accomplished after birth.

Money (1976) concludes that socialization is the main influence in individual gender differentiation because of the flexibility and interactive nature of even the biochemical components of sex differentiation. He offers the concept of *thresholds* which regulate the emergence of gender-related behavior:

> I prefer the concept of thresholds that facilitate or hinder the emergence and manifestation of given forms of behavior. I think the hormone–behavior story will eventually be told in terms of how hormones establish thresholds that regulate the ease or speed with which specified components or patterns of behavior manifest themselves, either spontaneously or in response to a stimulus. In this connection,

almost all behavioral sex differences will be understood not as absolutes, but as relative to the strength of the threshold that regulates their manifestation. In other words, most apparently sex-different behavior will actually be sex-shared, but threshold different. The exceptions relate to reproduction itself—impregnation in the male and menstruation, gestation, and lactation in the female. (p. 20)

Gender differences in behavior and attitudes are the result of the interaction of biological, social, and psychological influences. Even in individual cases of structural ambiguity in the body, it is impossible to clearly separate the differences between biological and social contributions. Our focus is on the social and psychological components. While we acknowledge the importance of hormonal influences on such gender-linked characteristics as aggression, we agree with Money that such characteristics are best understood as gender shared but threshold different.

Girls and boys grow up in different social and psychological environments, which influence their gender identity in decisive ways. Barry, Bacon, and Child (1957) reviewed data on socialization practices from anthropological studies of 110 cultures, most of which were nonliterate. Their data revealed that although differentiation of gender was not important in infancy, there were widespread patterns of reinforcing different behaviors in young girls and boys. Most cultures emphasized nurturance, obedience, and responsibility for girls, and self-reliance and achievement for boys. The researchers found that large gender differences in the socialization of girls and boys tended to be linked to large family systems and economies that valued physical strength and the superior development of motor skills. The authors concluded that in our society there was "relatively small sex differentiation" because of the value we place on intellectual rather than physical instrumentality.

The results of Block's (1973) cross-cultural study of differences in socialization practices in the United States, England, Sweden, Denmark, Finland, and Norway revealed that literate Western societies emphasize achievement, competition, control of feelings, and concern for conformity to rules for boys. The socialization of girls in the same societies stresses expression of feelings and physical affection, and the development of interpersonal relationships.

Williams (1974) and Maccoby and Jacklin (1974) reviewed studies of differences in gender-related behaviors and indicated how these differences contribute to gender identity. Following is a summary of the conclusions which were drawn from those two studies.

1. Behavioral differences between boy and girl neonates have not been conclusively demonstrated.

2. Absolute differences in cognitive ability and social behaviors in the first 2 years of life have not been conclusively demonstrated. Pat-

terning of cognitive development in girls is more strongly correlated with chronological age and with social class than it is for boys. Irritability and fearfulness are more consistently correlated with chronological age in boys.

3. In middle to late childhood, gender differences emerge as clear patterns in girls and boys. Girls show higher verbal aptitude. Spatial ability may be gender linked for boys.

4. Evidence for gender-linked differences in fearfulness, dependency, and nurturance is inconclusive. Teacher ratings and self-reports demonstrate that girls tend to be more fearful, but teachers' predispositions to assess these behaviors in girls, as well as girls' greater willingness to admit these feelings, may contribute to these findings. Girls seem more oriented toward interpersonal intimacy, but they do not necessarily exhibit more dependence behaviors. Both males and females can display nurturant play. Some evidence suggests that early exposure of males to infants and other small children enhances their nurturant behaviors as they mature.

5. From early childhood on, boys display a higher level of aggressive behavior than girls. This difference has been observed in both cross-cultural and animal studies. It is probable that the hormonal threshold for aggression in boys is "lower" or more "open" than in girls.

Socialization practices encourage gender-related behavior differences between boys and girls. Gender identity, as a concept related to self, is a scheme for the social categorization of individuals and includes a number of components. As Sherif (1982) points out, all known societies have some gender scheme through which the *meaning of biological differences* creates social roles or functions. Understanding an individual's knowledge of the categorical scheme for gender and her or his relationship to that scheme is as important as understanding the scheme itself.

Following a suggestion by Sherif, we use the terms *sex* and *gender* differently. *Sex* denotes structural biological differences and behaviors connected explicitly to those structural differences. *Gender* refers to the array of attributions and behaviors that concern identity or what it *means* to be male or female. The meaning of gender is complex and multileveled in adults.

The lack of distinction between sex and gender results in the tendency to consider behaviors such as aggression and nurturant responsiveness "sex different" and to overlook the social and psychological influences. Ullian (1981), for example, argues against "too hasty" a transformation of gender roles in our society due to differences in aggressiveness between boys and girls. She observes that young boys express their gender identity in more "exaggerated" ways than girls. She attributes this exaggeration to the identification of masculinity with degrees of physical prowess and size which are beyond the young boys' capacity. Ullian argues that boys must maximize the correspondence between their existing traits and the ideals they hold for masculinity in order to establish a secure male identity. The young girls, by contrast, express feminine attributes through smallness, dependence, and nurturance. According to Ullian, the young girl has available all that she needs to confirm her female identity—apart from the actual ability to reproduce. She concludes:

> If we seek to transform social roles in the direction of greater sexual equality, or increased androgyny, we must recognize that conceptions of masculinity and femininity are embedded in material more complex than adult directives and exhortations. To intercede more effectively, it is necessary to clarify for children the true distinguishing aspects of sexual gender—namely, the anatomical—and to emphasize their permanence, despite apparent changes suggested by clothing, physical appearance, social roles, and the like. Once this is accomplished, proper adult guidance and societal support may be more likely to enable the young child to proceed beyond that understanding to a fuller appreciation of the meaning and value of sexual equality. (p. 500)

Ullian's (1981) assumption that anatomical factors are the "true distinguishing aspects" of *gender* (rather than sex) is typical of some popular and psychoanalytic reasoning about male and female differences.

Chodorow (1978), by contrast, focuses her analysis on meaning rather than anatomy. In her view, anatomical differences between the sexes become symbolic representations of differences in social status and roles. Chodorow understands the girl's "envy" of a boy's penis, for example, as her envy of the greater independence and social privileges which appear to accrue to the boy from his having a penis. The penis thus symbolizes social privilege.

Research on early gender diferentiation certainly suggests that male gender identity is achieved later and with greater difficulty than female gender. Rather than conclude, however, that this is a result of the greater anatomical "distance" between the child and the adult male, we would argue from Chodorow's position that the absence of adult male caretakers in the growing boy's environment predisposes the boy to difficulties in achieving his male identity. Surrounded by powerful female figures at home and at school, the young boy develops his identity by excluding the feminine and imagining the masculine. From fantasy heroes and cartoon exaggerations of masculine prowess, young boys develop ideals for adult masculinity. Their exaggerated aggressive behavior can be understood as evolving from the absence of adult male role models and from the images of excessive power and strength that our culture conveys through its images of male heroes.

Both the superior social status of males and the absence of male caretakers contribute to difficulties for the young girl in the formation of her female gender identity. Although girls have many adult female role models to emulate, they must internalize inferior attributions about being weak, stupid, and dependent in order to establish their gender identity. The absence of validating male authority figures in the girl's daily environment predisposes her to develop a problematic "identity relationship" with her first male lover during her adolescence. She will project onto the young man the power to validate her goodness and worth—the power to "give" her self-esteem. The psychological development of female identity is far more complex than simply the struggle for male approval, however.

The first critical period for the development of female gender identity occurs between 18 months and 3 years of age. When the little girl identifies with being female, she assumes one of three adaptations: she becomes feminine and weak, masculine and strong, or feminine and strong (the traditional "father's daughter"). Each of these adaptations entails a loss. To be feminine and weak means thinking of oneself as inferior. To be masculine and strong means thinking of oneself as being "false," of having an adaptive cover over one's truly "flawed" nature. To be feminine and strong means thinking of oneself as maintaining a facade of self-reliance over a true identity of weakness and inferiority. At this early stage of her development, a girl may not experience identity conflict; later, however, an adult woman often imagines that she made some terrible mistake during this period. She imagines, for example, that she "needed too much" or was "too angry," or that she "covered up" some hidden flaw or emptiness.

The next critical period in the development of female identity is that of individuation from the family of origin during one's school years. When the girl moves into the outside world, she discovers more certainly that male activities and attitudes are valued over female ones. If the girl is healthy and basically secure she will opt either to "please" males with her appearance and achievements or to become "masculine" by identifying with males and their qualities. If the girl identifies herself as "inferior or weak," she can assume a posture of passive femininity without actively taking either of the male-adapted identity positions. When the girl makes the healthier adaptation of identifying with masculine ideals and attributes, she becomes increasingly aware that she has a "hidden" self of an underlying "inferiority" which she conceals by her adaptation. Under stress concerning her appearance or achievements, these girls can formulate a psychological rationale such as "I'm really stupid" or a physical rationale such as a psychosomatic ailment for their "hidden flaws."

The most critical period in a woman's early development is the separation from the family of origin which normally takes place in early adulthood. Conflicts in female identity are heightened at this time by the cultural emphasis on women's physical appearance and by the impossible "choices" the young woman faces. The woman's peers and family may formulate either–or choices such as family and marriage *or* independent career; an intimate relationship with a man *or* personal development. If the young woman consciously decides to "do both," the conflicting needs and demands of her roles will manifest themselves daily in her own and others' reflections. These are not merely private and personal inner conflicts; they are matters of "public concern" in that friends and neighbors will question the woman about "having a baby" or "going to graduate school" or about nursing her sick child or reporting to work. These either–or choices will result in an experience of loss which takes on a public character. Women cannot simply "leave behind" a career or mothering without being constantly questioned and examined about their choice.

In middle life, reevaluation of female identity confronts women with the constraints of their female gender. This reevaluation is feared by many women because they believe they have created a monster within. The woman may fear she is a "hag" or a wasted "has been" who must now face the loss of irretrievable opportunities. Or she may fear that she has become a lonely, constricted, and emotionally isolated "creature." Even when a woman in middle life experiences much satisfaction in her activities, she cannot avoid feeling that her identity as a woman is a "problem." Individuals fault themselves for having chosen wrongly in early life when, in fact, no choice could have resulted in a sense of completeness.

Finally, when a woman strives for the restoration of meaning in her later years, she must choose between understanding objectively the social constraints of her gender—which results in anger and resentment—and resigning herself to living through the achievements of her husband and children. Older women may reexperience the identity conflicts of earlier periods at this time, and the lack of their resolution will become a prominent concern.

In order to foster greater self-worth and internal validation in adult women, therapists and educators must acknowledge the conflicts inherent in female identity. Before we can aspire toward the ideal of androgyny, we must acknowledge what it means to be female in this period in our society. Whatever primary adaptation a woman may have developed—self-reliance or traditional femininity—she will inevitably experience inferiority and inadequacy in some of her daily contexts. Sherif (1982) says the following about conflict in female identity:

> There are problems of gender identity which can be conceptualized
> better as relationships among parts of the self-system, linked to dif-

ferent reference persons and groups. Such analysis suggests limitations to those conceptions of gender identity which do not deal with the devaluation of women but focus on the socially desirable traits in traditional stereotypes of women and men. . . . Newer conceptions appear to stress flexibility and adaptiveness, with little recognition that different parts of the self-system may conflict. To see one's self as both "independent" and "yielding," or as "defending own beliefs" and "gullible" can lead to considerable inner conflict, and can create havoc in one's personal relationships. . . . (p. 388)

Fragmentation of self and the demands of self-conflicting roles are constant themes for most adult women. These themes have little to do with immaturity or regression. The ideal of androgyny may accentuate conflict in a troubling way for an individual who is already aware of the conflicting role expectations within herself.

Androgyny is a combination of strong masculine and feminine traits. Bem, Martyna, and Watson (1976) have discovered that androgynous individuals of both sexes will display masculine independence and feminine nurture when the situation is appropriate for each kind of response. While this is certainly a meaningful ideal, many factors prevent its easy attainment.

Some mental health clinicians continue to consider the cluster of masculine identity traits "healthier" than androgyny (Kravetz & Jones, 1981). We can speculate that preference for masculine traits reflects the androcentric value we place on instrumentality and independence over and above interpersonal relatedness.

Gender identity conflict has been considered a symptom of undifferentiated gender in many mental illness syndromes. Strict adherence to gender attributes and roles appears to be an androcentric norm, as we have tried to demonstrate here. Conflict in gender identity in women, no matter what the individual's adaptation (i.e., as self-reliant, dependent, or androgynous), is to be expected as a result of female socialization within a patriarchal culture. Clarification of expected conflicts, and understanding of their relative adaptiveness for satisfactions in living, will enhance our ability to assist women in developing authority and competence.

FEMININE "NARCISSISM": ATTRACTING AND KEEPING A MAN

Women are often characterized, both in popular and in psychological contexts, as being preoccupied with appearance. Preoccupation with personal beauty has been analyzed as compensation for the missing penis, fear of achievement, inferior thinking, inferior physical strength, and/or lack of material resources. Women's narcissism is commonly thought to be a substitution for something more genuinely worthwhile. An extended analysis of feminine narcissism usually includes explanations of women's efforts to attract and "trap" men, and their ability to be gratified vicariously through the achievements of husbands or children. Because of ambivalent feelings about vicarious gratifications, the woman theoretically also fears that she will lose her beauty, youth, and slender body when she assumes the role of wife and mother. Pregnancy is interpreted in most psychoanalytic theories as presenting a serious challenge to a woman's narcissism: Can the woman translate her narcissistic needs to be beautiful and cherished into giving the "gift of life" to others? Pregnancy and childbirth are thus considered critical tasks in the woman's maturation.

In one study (Devereux, 1960), the female "castration complex" was related to female narcissism on the basis of an examination of male fantasies, cross-cultural historical references, and 17 cases in psychotherapy. The finding that woman view themselves as inferior and their genitals as repugnant was understood in terms of their anxieties concerning fantasies of castration (i.e., of having lost a penis through some unknown fault of their own). To compensate for their loss, women were considered to reassure themselves through sexual foreplay that they were still attractive and that their genitals did not repel their male partners.

Theories of feminine narcissism fail to account for the social context in which a woman's appearance is the only socially condoned form of power openly afforded her. As Chernin (1981) has articulated in her analysis of women's preoccupations with slenderness, an attractive body image is a socially condoned form of competition for women. Encouraged by our friends, partners, parents, associates, and the media, we compete for social power by seeking to be more beautiful than other women.

Nowhere are the destructive effects of this competition more obvious than in the eating disorders. In their study of anorexia and bulimia in women, Wooley and Wooley (1980) trace the social and cultural pressures concerning food, eating, and appearance in women's lives. They note that having a slender and attractive appearance is a prerequisite for entrance into a number of women's professions (e.g., airline attendant). Women accrue both interpersonal and material rewards from their preoccupation with appearance, and they stand to lose relationships, income, self-esteem, and peer approval (not to mention dates with men) if they "let go" of their hold on their appearance. Women's self-esteem is understandably tied directly to their body image.

If a woman survives the "narcissistic shock" of pregnancy and the changes in body image, what are her social and psychological rewards?

While the institution of motherhood is idealized in our society, it carries little social or symbolic power. All the same, Americans make a common assumption that a mother is responsible, even solely responsible, for the psychological and physical welfare of her children. If something goes awry in their development, she is often blamed. This social condition has aptly been called "powerless responsibility" by Rich (1976).

Women have been blamed for not "giving enough" to their children's emotional development or for giving in the wrong way. Many years ago, Horney (1933) described the mother as the major source of pathology in the disturbance of children. That a mother foists her unhappiness and unresolved fears onto her children is familiar popular wisdom. Confusing and poorly conceived communications from mothers have been called the "primary toxic agent" in schizophrenia (Goldfarb, Goldfarb, & Scholl, 1966). Mother herself has been labeled "schizophrenogenic" and faulted for her hostile and destructive love. The mother–daughter relationship has been the focus for psychiatric understanding of eating disorders, with the quality of the mother's "overinvolvement" often blamed for the child's disease.

Although women are presumed to mature and develop in their roles of wife and mother, the actual effects of these roles on women's health and well-being appear to be contrary to theory. Bernard (1972) presents an impressive argument that marriage benefits husbands more than wives and that single women are healthier than married women. Supporting evidence for her argument comes from her finding asymmetries between men and women on a wide range of indices including psychological distress, mental health impairment, physical health, income, crime, suicide, and alcoholism. In another study, Gove (1972) reviewed the relationship between marital status and mental health in industrial societies since World War II. While married men and women had lower rates of mental illness than the unmarried of both sexes, married women reported more disturbances than married men.

The actual effects of marriage and mothering on the life satisfactions of adult women have not been broadly studied until quite recently. Baruch, Barnett, and Rivers (1983) report the results of a very informative study of patterns of work and relationship among more than 300 American women in the age range of 35 to 55. Their results strongly support the thesis that challenging paid work, accompanied by supportive egalitarian relationships with men, contributes most strongly to a woman's sense of well-being in adult life. They comment that the role of stay-at-home childrearing may be today's "high-risk" occupation. Married women, unemployed and at home with children, reported higher levels of dissatisfaction and distress than any other group except unemployed married women at home with no children.

Our idealization of motherhood and self-sacrifice has obscured our understanding of the psychological effects of powerless responsibility. Psychological theories of selfless love and feminine narcissism share an androcentric connection in the belief that women mature and achieve satisfaction by sacrificing their self-interest. This is not to imply that nurturing and caregiving are inferior activities, but only that they need to be chosen in and of themselves in order to be satisfying. When a woman pursues female power through appearance, she is led to believe that rewards for her beautiful appearance will come through the roles of wife and mother. These roles result in powerless responsibility rather than social power. Adolescent women especially are at risk for believing cultural stereotypes about female beauty as power. As psychotherapists, we must increasingly become aware of the actual social meanings associated with the power of female appearance and whether or how they bring real satisfaction.

FEMININE "MASOCHISM": EMBRACING SUFFERING

Since Deutsch published her two-volume *Psychology of Women* in 1944 and 1945, her ideas have influenced many psychiatric theories about women's identity. Deutsch contended that the essential characteristic of the adult woman's personality was "masochism," or the willingness to embrace suffering. Since a woman's life necessarily involved suffering through menstruation, pregnancy, childbirth, menopause, and sacrifices for others, a woman must learn to adjust and submit to pain.

Deutsch (1944, 1945) contended, further, that every aspect of a woman's identity is colored by her ability to accept and even love the pain related to her biology and inherent social roles. Many psychiatric studies and interventions concerning women's pain have focused on the idea that we must accept suffering or fail to be fully female. Benedek (1959) provided a good case study of masochism as the essence of female identity. Noting that girls are introduced through menstruation to painful female suffering, Benedek asserted that the sooner a girl can accept the discomfort of her monthly cycle as a normal part of her experience, the better prepared she will be for the next pain involved with loss of virginity. These early discomforts of her adult female biology only set the stage for the later sacrifices she must make in caring for her husband and children.

The blending of pain and satisfaction in the theory of feminine masochism has resulted in confusion both for women and for therapists who counsel them. Women's painful experiences with their reproductive systems have been interpreted as ambivalence toward the demands of adult femininity and fearful anticipation of the pains of childbirth.

Curious as it may seem, the psychiatric literature since Deutsch has been replete with psychogenic explanations for women's reproductive distress. Vomiting in pregnancy, infertility, "frigidity" in sexual responses, fears of childbirth, and menstrual discomfort have all been understood as women's ambivalence about assuming the suffering inherent in their feminine roles.

This view has some truth, of course, since anyone would fear pain, especially the kind of unpredictable pain caused by some reproductive conditions. Concluding that *women's* fear of pain arises from an unwillingness to accept their femininity results in paradoxically blaming the victim for her condition. Rather than responding with an empathy which acknowledges the reality of reproductive stresses in women's lives, many clinicians have responded as if the woman's ambivalence actually created the distress.

The following examples are representative of many studies of female masochism. Benedek (1952) published an article which considered infertility a "psychosomatic defense" which can be interpreted as the woman's unconscious anxiety about motherhood. Chertok, Mondzain, and Bonnaud (1963) interpreted vomiting in pregnancy as an expression of the ambivalence felt by the woman toward the fetus. The ambivalence was thought to derive from the mother's lack of acceptance of the responsibility of female adulthood. Levitt and Lubin (1967) reported results from administering personality scales and correlating them with complaints about menstruation. They found that women's complaints were "related to an unwholesome menstrual attitude" and to neurotic and paranoid tendencies. In the 1950s (e.g., Harvey & Sherfey, 1954), a countertrend began to develop regarding the "pain" of women's reproductive systems. Warnings were made about using overly simplistic psychodynamic explanations for events that could have physiological or more complicated psychophysiological bases. Emerging from medical persuasions opposed to psychoanalysis was the idea that women should be more like men: They should simply ignore the minor stresses of their reproductive biology.

Only recently have we come out from under the weight of androcentric reasoning about psychobiological aspects of women's psychology. The masochistic psychology of compensation (for the missing penis) initially interfered with helping women respond actively to reproductive and hormonal stresses. Then the masculine psychology of "grin and bear it" imposed a strictly male orientation toward fluctuating emotional states: They were said to be a "figment of imagination."

Contemporary studies of women's menstrual cycles demonstrate more objectively what Deutsch (1944) and Benedek (1952, 1959) were intuitively struggling toward in the miasma of the femininity of their time: Affect in women *is* closely related to levels of hormonal production. A realistic female self-concept needs to include conscious recognition of the psychology of the hormonal cycle both over a lifetime and within the menstrual period itself. Premenstrual syndrome is a period of hormonal stress during which many women tend to experience lowered self-esteem and feelings of helplessness, anger, fear, and anxiety. These hormonal effects have been well documented in both cross-sectional and longitudinal studies (e.g, Dalton, 1964; Ivey & Bardwick, 1968; Parlee, 1973). During the period of time between ovulation and menstural bleeding, women can expect certain fluctuations in their affective states that may increase their need for warmth, support, and affection. The fluctuations in mood do not tend to influence activity in significant ways, however, when menstruating women are compared to men or nonmenstruating women (Dan, 1976). Accommodation and planning in recognition of the potential for mood fluctuation can assist women in maintaining self-esteem and comfort through the more stressful period of the monthly menstrual cycle.

Studies of pregnancy (e.g., Shereshefsky, 1970) and menopause demonstrate that these normal physiological events signal both developmental transitions and special affective states that must be considered in women's psychology. Emotional turmoil often occurs with both of these events, but it does not need to be disruptive and can, in fact, be a positive influence on our self-concepts and self-esteem.

While reproductive health for women is composed of a different set of variables than for men, we have no evidence from our work or from the studies we have reviewed, that anxiety about self-concept arises directly from hormonal or reproductive stresses. Rather, it seems to arise from the self-blame and self-hatred that women experience when they attempt to constrain themselves to fit the ideals of masochism or masculinity.

FEMININE "PASSIVITY": DEPENDING ON MEN

Women continue to encounter the idealization of passivity as a life-style and a mode of feminine behavior. Sometimes the most difficult encounter is with our mothers, who understandably want to justify their choices of dependent life-styles. On an everyday basis, girls and women are often instructed to wait for what they want, whether that means dates with men, praise from a superior, or educational goals. Many women are confused by the value our society places on passivity for females, and may be even further confused by the recent advocating of "receptivity" that is part of some feminist critiques of our culture. Notably, passivity and receptivity are two different psychological states, but many of us are not clear about the differences. *Passivity* is inactivity and unresponsiveness, a simple waiting to be fulfilled. *Receptivity* is activity and responsively waiting for the right moment to connect to one's desire. Passivity involves taking no prespective while receptivity involves choice and insight.

The notion that women are inherently passive derives from the idea that they are inferior. Because the woman is childlike, weaker, less intelligent, etc., she must be protected and guided by men and her elders. From classical psychoanalysis, we are offered the explanation that girls fail to internalize a rational and principled morality because they cannot completely identify with their mothers, who do not have penises.

From a cultural point of view, women are socialized to be emotionally and materially dependent on men so that they can be "kept" at home to specialize in caregiving and childrearing. In the last three decades of American society, socialization toward economic dependency in females has been based on the assumption of the family wage system. As Ehrenreich (1983) has indicated in her study of men's roles, the family wage system is rapidly disappearing, and men are happy to relinquish the role of sole breadwinner. In the meantime, however, girls continue to be socialized toward passive dependence.

Identifying with traditionally masculine attitudes of independence and action seems to be a healthier adaptation for girls, however, than identifying with feminine passivity. In a longitudinal follow-up study of middle childhood, Sears (1970) found that a traditional feminine identity in childhood was associated with poor self-concept, aggression, and anxiety in adulthood. Williams (1974) discovered in her study of adolescent girls that identification with "dominant–ascendant" attitudes of the father led to higher levels of personal adjustment. Adolescent girls who identified with their mothers' more passive attitudes were less well adjusted. Heilbrun (1968) also found that girls who were assessed as "better adjusted" on psychological measures were more masculine in self-concept than other girls. Masculine girls are described by these investigators as having better coping skills; being more goal oriented, more instrumental in their own lives; and as more expressive than their feminine counterparts.

Ehrenreich (1983) articulates the social bind of women's material dependence on men. Women have had no clear claim on men's wages over these past three decades, yet most women have been confined to the home. Men have been free to support or not support their wives and children, while women have had to rely on good faith, a position of considerable anxiety and insecurity.

From the research done by Baruch *et al.* (1983) on well-being in women's adult life, we would conclude that material (economic) dependence and career incompetence are the greatest threats to the psychological welfare of females in our society. However the ideals of passivity are fashioned—whether as a form of the "Cinderella complex" (Dowling, 1981) or as a nostalgia for the "feminine mystique"—these ideals collide with the fact that material dependence in adulthood is psychologically stressful, often leading to depression and alcohol abuse, and inevitably accompanied by low self-esteem.

A major developmental achievement of early adulthood is the ability to distinguish between material and emotional dependence. This distinction is realized through the material independence of the adult child, who can then return home with the freedom to love and to be loved as a person. Both the grown child and the parents clarify their emotional needs for each other in this rapprochment after separation. When women transfer their economic dependence directly from parents to husband, they miss the opportunity to distinguish between these two kinds of dependence. This missed opportunity can result in severe insecurity about leaving home, the condition called "agoraphobia."

The agoraphobic woman cannot distinguish the boundaries of her dependence. She experiences herself as excessively helpless, frequently in a "collapsed" state. In essence, the woman finds herself in the position of a grown child staying with parents; she is insecure in her ability to sustain herself as an individual. Such a woman has not recognized the difference between emotional and material dependence.

The pressure to conform to an adult identity that includes passivity as a central feature is anxiety provoking in itself. Studies of adults using Rotter's (1966) "locus of control" measure of self-agency support the idea that passivity and dependence are stressful components of self-image. Studies have demonstrated that American women are more "external" in their orientation than are American men (e.g., Brannigan & Tolor, 1971). Women are more passive toward their fate; that is, they expect that forces "out there" have more determining effects on their lives than they do themselves. The opposite orientation, "internal locus of control," has been found to be positively related to greater personal adjustment, higher self-esteem, and a greater sense of self-determination.

The constrictions of traditional feminine gender identity are greatest in adolescence, when young women are initially confronting choices concerning partnership with a man. As Douvan (1970) discovered, young women suffer more from the stringent imposition of gender typing than do older women. Adolescent girls continue to be misled into believing they can fulfill their identity needs by becoming materially dependent. These girls are at risk for developing what we call an "identity relationship" with the boy or man "of their dreams." In such a situation, the girl wholly identifies with the values, goals, and personal orientation of the man, anxiously projecting her identity needs onto him. She believes that she will be fulfilled in living through his success and achievements, and in being protected by his greater strength, wealth or intelligence. Awareness of the deleterious effects of idealized passivity should help psychotherapists assist young women in distinguishing between authentic needs for emotional dependence and wishful preoccupations with passive dependence.

In order to distinguish between patriarchal ideals for material dependence and female strengths of emotional interdependence, we need an accurate language. We prefer to use the term *passivity* to indicate the attitude of passive dependence and vicarious identification with others' successes. The word *dependence* can then be freed of some of its pejorative load and recognized as a basic emotional need in human life, central to survival.

Understanding a certain style of dependence to be an ideal for human life, we have chosen the concept of *empathy* to express this ideal. As Jordan (1983) says, ''In order to empathize, one must have a well-differentiated sense of self in addition to an appreciation of and sensivity to the differentness as well as the sameness of another person'' (p. 2).

Empathy involves a complex set of interpersonal variables which center around interest in another, identification with the other, and awareness of one's own individuality.

Some psychological theories of development have confused empathy with passivity, symbiosis, sympathy, regression, and even merging of self and other. Differentiating empathy as a developmental achievement will assist us in helping women distinguish between interdependent sensitivity and the propensity to surrender one's will. As Jordan (1983) points out, females have been found to be more empathic than males in research done on various constructs of empathy. According to Jordan, further: ''Problems with empathy for females . . . typically involve difficulty reinstating a sense of self and cognitively structuring the experience'' (p. 3). In other words, some women have difficulty in actively moving out of affective identification and using language to depict what happened. In order to increase their potentials for true empathy, women may need to oppose their socialized tendency to surrender their individuality in the face of another's emotional needs or demands.

Ideals of passive dependency and notions of inherent passivity in females must be actively opposed in order to increase female authority. At the same time, empathy and interdependence can be differentiated as potential strengths to be developed out of female socialization.

3

Basic Considerations: Competence, Feminism, and Jung

As women, we are often reticent to trust in the strength of our own experience, especially when it is challenged by powerful males and masculine standards for truth, beauty, or goodness. We have in fact been socialized to believe that we lack something and that we are thus destined never to rightfully fill the decision-making positions of symbolic authority in our society. Many of us say to ourselves privately, if not publicly, "I must be doing something wrong because look how I have failed (with my children, my educational goals, whatever)." We have internalized a deficit orientation toward ourselves and find that a focus on our strengths or competences is uncomfortable if not alien. We resist the idea that we are capable, intelligent, and strong because our self-concept has been organized around its opposite. Acknowledging our strengths leads to anxiety.

Many times in counseling male–female couples we have heard something like the following interchange:

SHE: I feel so exhausted from running around after the kids and picking up around the house.
HE: You couldn't be tired. You slept until noon today and I got breakfast for the kids. You don't even hold a job.
SHE: I guess you're right. I couldn't be tired. Maybe I'm depressed.

The essential element here is that the woman abandons the validity of her own perspective that she is tired. Once she has given up on her idea, she readily takes on a deficit view of herself (that she is depressed).

Our therapeutic orientation toward increasing competence and strengths has led us to a confrontation with many ordinary assumptions of everyday life, especially as they have been internalized by

28

women. Consequently, we need to clarify some of our terms and theoretical assumptions. This chapter is our attempt to claim the validity of our approach and to explicate our framework from a nondeficit perspective. This means that we will not defend our orientation elaborately, but rather we will try to present it on its own terms.

First, we define *competence* as a vital connection to one's life and circumstances. It is a feeling of being in control (perceived control), of being capable of active encounter with one's conditions of living. Everyone who has lived beyond 2 days in the complex interactive organic system of the human body has developed adaptive strengths. Certainly by the time the organism has matured enough to be called a "person"— reliably around 18 months or so—an individual has many strengths and abilities for active manipulation, cognitive evaluation and anticipation, and communicative involvement with both the physical and human environments.

As physically weak animals, we are enormously dependent on other members of our species. Consequently we develop elaborate communication skills that preoccupy us, dominating our interests for the entire life cycle. We are social animals. The human "body" is the social group, and many of our adaptive strengths are organized around symbolic expression and contact with each other. Any person who walks into our offices is competent at many complex forms of communication or that person would not have survived.

To reiterate, women are reluctant and anxious about claiming their competences. Internalized feelings of inferiority result in anxiety about one's strengths. Initially when we attend to strengths and competences in assessment, women clients make a constant effort to convince us otherwise. The debilitating preoccupation with low self-esteem emerges in transitory identifications with fear, jealousy, aggression, depression, anxiety, and helplessness. Many women are afraid that they are not capable of doing what will be asked of them, and they imagine that what is being asked concerns perfect accommodation to someone else's (e.g., the therapist's) needs or demands. After clients understand their own propensity to blame themselves and to focus on deficits, it is not difficult to form a lasting rapport around the project of combating internalized oppression.

Before we elaborate our methods of assessment and assumptions about therapy, we would like to introduce the clients we see in our practices. We are both currently in independent practice of psychotherapy. We are certified Jungian analysts, self-declared feminist therapists, and licensed psychologists. One of us (Young-Eisendrath) is also a certified (ACSW) social worker. We have general practices of psychotherapy, sometimes conducting Jungian analysis and sometimes doing other forms of counseling and therapy. We have more than 20 years of combined experience during which each of us has worked in public clinics and mental health facilities, and taught in graduate schools (psychology and social work) in addition to our current independent practices.

PRESENTING PROBLEMS AMONG CONTEMPORARY WOMEN

In order to clarify some of the generational differences in the problems which our adult clients present to us, we will review some major sociological themes that characterize the women in our practice.

Women who are now in their 20s and early 30s appear at our doors with complaints that we could broadly characterize as the residue of the recent turmoil in the women's movement. They have intense identity conflicts, largely conscious, about ''what they should do with their lives.'' They feel pressure to have a career and pressure to have a family. With the recent influx of skepticism about the possibility of ''doing it all,'' they are convinced that they have to make a choice. Often they have grown up wanting a career, but are already tired of competing for rewards in school or elsewhere that do not seem financially promising or existentially satisfying. The professions are crowded, graduate schools are overenrolled, and the traditional roles of wife and mother look comforting to them.

Women in their middle 30s and 40s approach us still in the throes of the women's movement and other broad ethical issues. They have strong social values, commitment to humanitarian ideals and antimaterialism, and a host of other ''pro-and-anti'' concerns which they may or may not have been able to differentiate. Often they have taken what Erikson (1968) called a ''moratorium'' on adulthood and have escaped into some aspect of their early idealism. In deficit language, they may be said to have an ''identity disorder'' of adolescence in adulthood. They feel jaded and bitter about how misled they were by promises of autonomy and relationships with men. They may have become lesbian in the process of evaluating heterosexual relating. They may or may not have ''made it'' in the work environment of their choice, but they are typically facing some kind of new hurdle (e.g., advanced training, tenure review, advancement on the job) that they consider the ultimate test of their worth, skills, or competence. Often they have given up on men, especially men in their own generation, whom they find inaccessible, uncommitted, too traditional, or otherwise separate from themselves. They may or may not have children, but the maternal identity they rejected earlier is now emerging and they are concerned about how to relate again to the ''idea of having babies.'' Many of these women are not in settled couple relationships, and they are involved in, or are considering the pros and cons of single parenting.

Women in their middle 40s and 50s more often than not appear with concern of identity transition. They have been wives and mothers, volunteers, and PTA leaders; now they want to know what to do with their lives. They may be motivated to return to work or school, or they may not be so motivated, but either way, they are typically afraid. They fear abandonment by their husbands, children, and even friends. Their self-esteem is especially low, and they frequently show signs that they feel unable to become authoritative adults. Most prominent to them is the problem of their "stupidity." They believe that their minds have "gone bad" during the years of mothering and caregiving, and that they are not able to compete with younger women, whom they see as more competent, freer, and more able to be satisfied with their lives. To some extent, these older women are contemptuous or skeptical about younger women, especially those who seem vitally engaged with life.

Finally, women in their late 50s and 60s who arrive at our offices often seem the most hopeless. Many have been abandoned, some after years in primarily caregiving roles, and now they are depressed and bitter. They have suffered from some or all of the "5 D's": death, disease, divorce, desertion, and drunkenness. At the beginning, their contempt for life and their despair seem overwhelming, and suicide emerges most forcefully as a real and meaningful consideration as they face existential questions about identity choices and adaptations, which have, in their experience, been controlled by forces outside themselves.

Through all of these themes some motifs regularly repeat. The first is trouble with food, eating, or drinking, and with body image. Women of all ages worry about their eating habits, their weight, and their appearance. The so-called eating disorders are prevalent among all of our clients, who recognize consciously or unconsciously, that appearance is socially condoned power (Wooley & Wooley, 1980). Without a beautiful appearance, or some approximation of it, a woman realistically fears a frightening drop in self-esteem. Eating disorders are actually interpersonal identity concerns, which must be solved at the level of interpersonal relating and of understanding the symbolic meanings of food and body. Our approach does not exclude work on behaviors, but it begins with questions about a woman's ideal self rather than ideal weight.

The second motif is that of a "basic flaw" or "hidden" ugliness, stupidity, or meanness. All of our clients have "secrets" which involve self-condemnation and seeing themselves as bad or flawed. The flaw may take the form of physical or psychological defects, low scores on intelligence tests, or "sinful" or "wicked" behavior. We have never encountered a woman in therapy who did not believe she was hiding a secret flaw that others would eventually discover.

Finally, there is often fear concerning financial security, even among

the wealthiest of women. Most of our clients worry about their security in material terms and confuse financial security with emotional security. The process of realistically sorting out the dimensions of the two
is an exercise in increasing self-control, if not self-esteem.

In order to set the stage for the conceptual framework we will build,
we want to turn our attention specifically to the problem of assessment.
How can we approach our clients without aggravating their deficit
thinking and despair?

ASSESSING COMPETENCE IN CONTEXT

To replace the deficit model of psychopathology, we use a frame of
reference that is systematic and adequate to the task of assessing both
a person's current life difficulties and ongoing strengths. We are familiar with many other efforts to do something similar (e.g., Miller, 1976;
Bond & Rosen, 1980). Working within a community of thinkers, we offer our ideas in the spirit of a common project to develop an alternative
model of assessment. Our approach integrates the contributions of
Loevinger (1976), Albee and Joffe (1977), and feminist therapists (Brodsky & Hare-Mustin, 1980) with Jung's psychology in assessing symbolic meaning, psychological development, immediate interpersonal
relating, and the larger social context. These elements are cast in the
framework of competence. Because our sphere of concern is complex—
that is, understanding the meaning and motivational aspects of interpersonal human relating—our reference system is also rather complex. Our
combined focus on relationships, cultural and social influences (both
in the immediate environment and in the dominant society), and symbolic expression (in behavior and dreams) is difficult to manage at times,
but will, we hope, eventually be streamlined as we modify our framework. We restrain our predisposition to focus on "less than" characteristics in our clients (e.g., weaker, less assertive, less powerful,
poorer), but we are also the products of our culture. Sometimes we still
fall into the prevailing cultural stereotypes.

The skeletal frame of our model of assessment is described below.

Assess Competence

Our definition of competence includes the subset of *coping* or dealing
successfully with ongoing and past environmental demands for effective
action, but we define competence more fully in terms of identity: the
recognized elements of a person's effectiveness as an actor in her life.
Whereas coping may be entirely unconscious (e.g., joining a religious

group as a way of getting out of the house), competence includes awareness of one's own strengths. How does this person include a sense of competence in her attitude about her life situation? In what areas of life does she act with the knowledge that she is an effective agent? What situations offer promise for building competence, such as improving her skills through further education or validating her accomplishments with pay or appreciation?

Assess Vulnerabilities

In what ways is this person vulnerable to loss of self-esteem or reduced effectiveness of action? Included as a central issue here is gender identity: How much has a woman identified with being weak, stupid, powerless, dependent, irrational, or excessively emotional? Internalizing these attributions can make her too vulnerable to interpersonal stimuli, and render her especially sensitive to what family members and friends say about her personal qualities. Similarly, physical illness, poverty, aging, and disability are vulnerabilities that can interfere with her sense of competence and her ability to lead a useful life. Some vulnerabilities must be accepted and planned for (e.g., diabetes), whereas others can be worked through and discarded (e.g, the idea of inferiority connected to female gender). Regardless of the source, a vulnerability is recognized specifically by a long-term tendency toward feeling defeated or hopeless.

Some severe psychological vulnerabilities arise when trying to reach a consensus about the reality of perceptions and cognitions, that is, about the reality of one's own experience in the context of others' experience. If early family relationships were especially burdened with conflict, and environmental circumstances were disruptive, a person can become vulnerable to the confusing of symbolic and emotional reality with literal and concrete reality. Even such severe vulnerabilities, however, can be understood as both meaningful and hopeful, as indicating "where to go" or how to develop further. Jung's psychology, especially, prompts us to ask "What is the meaning of this particular weakness and how can it be used as a strength?"

Assess Stresses

Stress is understood in terms of critical life factors which currently require special adaptive responses in the person's life. Stressful events include life transitions (e.g., giving birth, changing residences, returning to school), acute physical illnesses (chronic illness would be a vulnerability), and other similar situations currently relevant. Stresses and vulnerabilities may overlap. For instance, vulnerability to attributions about being stupid may arise during a particularly stressful situation in a school classroom, or out of a difficult relationship with an authority figure at work.

We have not found it necessary to quantify our assessments in any of these areas. We find descriptive language, which cites examples and quotations from a client's life situation, precise enough to assist us in formulating appropriate goals and tasks for therapy.

Because of the imposition of the medical model on most forms of psychotherapy (due in part to insurance companies insisting on deficit diagnoses for reimbursements), the competence approach surprises many clients. Discussion about current strengths and the possibility of expanding them can be uplifting, providing it is not too confusing to a person habituated to thinking in terms of deficits only.

Several structural developmental models (e.g., Piaget's [1926] cognitive development; Loevinger's [1976] ego development; and Kohlberg's [1981] moral development, as revised for women by Gilligan, 1982) help us study the process of human development more intensively and systematically than we could have previously in psychotherapy. Although Jung (1969b) offered the first formal psychological conception of life-span development with his idea of integrating unconscious complexes over a lifetime, he did not extrapolate or explore the idea explicitly enough to make it a match for categories of psychopathology.

Current object relations theorists, beginning with Klein (1932) and Sullivan (1953), add theories of affective development that introduce greater precision in describing emotional, symbolic communications. Structural developmental models and affective theories are underpinnings for the model we use to assess competence, vulnerability, and stress in women's functioning.

As a competence model is made more precise and systematic, it can be offered as a replacement for the symptomatic descriptions that deficit thinking imposes on interpersonal assessment. Until such a transition is complete, however, we believe that it is incumbent on feminist therapists to be familiar with the deficit language of psychopathology—for example, the third edition of the *Diagnostic and Statistical Manual of Mental Disorders* (American Psychiatric Association, 1980)—in order to be informed critics in the psychological community. Consequently, we will include this language in some of our descriptions, while we emphasize that it is not our frame of reference.

Finally, emphasizing competence opens up a new understanding of the therapeutic relationship. If the client is not sick, then she should be engaging in life while in therapy, through both work and interpersonal relationships. Whether the work is paid or not, and this includes housework and schoolwork, it should be recognized and appreciated.

Therapy is a transitory relationship of a particular nature, with formal roles and a nonpersonal, consultative type of ritual. Ever since Freud's contributions to the understanding of transference, therapists have acknowledged their own responsibility for finding meaningful, intimate relationships outside of therapy so as not to confuse their own personal needs with those of their clients. We believe that it is also the therapist's responsibility not to allow the client to take a moratorium on life while in therapy or to become overly dependent on the therapist. We have seen women clients, in particular, who have spent years in analysis maintaining a quasi-dating posture with their analysts. Although no actual sexual or personal contact may have been made, the promise lingered for the client, partly because she was seen as sick, dependent, or incapable, while her therapist was by definition an authority, an expert, and an independent agent. In some cases, an even more complicated situation would ensue in which the client would return repeatedly to therapy in an unconscious attempt to "cure" the therapist who seemed hopelessly depressed. Such a situation is due, in part, to the severely impoverished interpersonal relationship that the therapist offered the client. Perhaps some kind of healing can take place under these conditions, but it would be ambiguous at best. If a client continues for years in a therapy relationship that is the central, most involved, and most intimate interpersonal relationship in the client's life then generally there is a problem inherent in the therapy.

Viewing the client as a partner in a collaborative process, to which the therapist brings specialized psychological knowledge, responsibility, techniques, and information, results in less risk that the client will use therapy as a place to hide from life rather than as a place to learn more about engaging it. Recognizing the client's competence also helps to prevent the therapist from leaning on the client's "illness" for the therapist's financial or emotional needs. Psychotherapists can function quite usefully, and analytically, in the role that was once that of the family doctor: that is, as a servant to the needs of the client. The client comes at times of crisis, breakdown, or reorganization of personality. The therapist consults and works with the client to try out new activities, attitudes, and possibilites in the interpersonal context of the client's life, even with clients who need regular, ongoing, and frequent consultation for extended periods of time.

A FEMINIST APPROACH TO JUNG'S PSYCHOLOGY

We use Jung's (e.g., 1969a) ideas of complex, archetype, persona, animus/anima, and individuation both in clinical interpretations and in conceptualizing women's development. We believe that Jung's (e.g., 1966) psychology offers a unique method of interpretation, among the psychodynamic methods, for preserving the imagistic character of nonrational expressions (in dreams, symbols, creative work, and interpersonal relating). Jung did not reduce the nonrational to a causal or historical explanation expressed in a rational sentence; instead, he expanded the meaning of an image or gesture by referring it to similar images from mythology, ritual, art, or literature, thus situating the individual in relation to the archaic and enduring aspects of human reality.

In order to use Jung's psychology with feminist therapy, we have revised and systematized some of his concepts. We believe our revisions to be consistent with Jung's (1969a) own revision of his work during the latter part of his life, from about 1935 to 1961, when he had become acquainted with ethological studies and modern biology. At the time, he distinguished between the archetype as form and the culturally influenced archetypal images which are expressed in motifs that allude to an underlying common form.

We find several of Jung's revolutionary contributions to psychotherapy to be compatible with feminist therapy and to expand some of the principles which are currently identified as feminist by contributors to the literature. First, Jung (1966) emphasized *reconstructing the current conscious attitude* in psychotherapy, rather than recovering or uncovering the historical past. From a feminist perspective, we assist our clients in an ongoing examination of their assumptions about themselves in a social context, and especially their unconscious assumptions regarding female gender identity. Jung wrote in 1929 that "neurosis or any other mental conflict depends much more on the personal attitude of the patient than on his infantile history" (1966, p. 31). This focus on the present and actual attitude directs primary therapeutic consideration in the personal, in the context of the client's immediate interpersonal relationships (including the therapeutic relationship), and to current concerns relevant to her position in the life cycle.

Just as feminist therapy assumes a model of collaboration for the work of therapy, also Jung conceived of the work of analysis as a mutual endeavor between analyst and analysand, in which the analyst should be influenced and changed through the process as she or he assists the analysand in changing. In 1929 Jung wrote: "the doctor is as much 'in the analysis' as the patient. He is equally a part of the psychic process of treatment and therefore equally exposed to the transforming influences" (1966, p. 72). This was a revolutionary idea then and still is. Psychoanalytic reformers such as Langs and Searles (1980) have recently discovered this same effect on the therapist. Schafer's (1983) model for the psychoanalytic life history is a narrative construction, which is mutually influenced through the shared participation of analyst and analysand.

Jung's (1969b) idea of a psychological *complex* relates to these therapeutic methods of meaning reconstruction and collaboration of therapist and client. As in Jung's theory, we define a complex as a collection of images, ideas, feelings, and habitual actions that is compelling or motivating in a nonrational way. A complex in interpersonal relating is experienced as a habitual field of action, symbol, and emotion organized around a core state of emotional arousal. This core state concerns a typical aspect of human life. Examples of ordinary complexes of everyday living are "I," Mother,[1] Father, Child, and anima/ animus. Complexes are not rationally discrete entities, but are emotional states of being which are enacted in typical ways. Some complexes are conscious, or partly conscious, and familiar. The body-image complex organized around the experience of "I" is at least partly conscious in most adults. Some complexes, however, are wholly unconscious. The complex organized around the excluded aspects of one's gender identity, the *animus complex* in a woman, is typically unconscious until it is interpreted and analyzed. An unconscious complex may be projected onto someone else, or it may be momentarily identified with and taken on as an alien attitude. When an unconscious complex overtakes one's conscious identity, the person feels "beside herself" with strange moods, anxieties, and ideas. In order for such a "possession" by a complex to continue in an interpersonal field, somebody else usually has to pick up and enact a role that fits into the complex. A person may also experience inner conflict between complexes. Usually there is a conflict between one's current conscious attitude and a less conscious complex. There may be, for example, conflict between one's moral judgment and an urge to act in opposition to it.

According to Jung's (1969a) psychology, the reason that a complex is so compelling and so difficult to manage intentionally is that it is organized around an archetype. Consistent with Jung's (1969a) definition of *archetype as such*, we use the term to mean a universal tendency to respond to a typical human situation of instinctual–emotional arousal

1. We use lowercase letters to refer to actual persons, such as mother and father. A capitalized noun referring to these roles (Mother, Father, Alien Outsider) refers to the psychological complex—the core of which is archetypal—as experienced within an individual or constellated in an interpersonal field of communication.

by forming affective images. The images correspond to emotional arousal in a relationship. The relationship may be between complexes (e.g., the Mother complex vs. one's conscious attitude) or between people (e.g., the actual mother vs. myself). Jung's idea of the archetype as an organizing pattern for the expression of human instinctual/emotional responses is similar to Bowlby's (1969) concept of human instinct.

Jung and Bowlby agree that human instincts are not simple, spontaneous impulses, but are patterned behaviors, which emerge only in particular relational contexts for which they have been programmed. These social or relational instincts have become centrally built into the species for survival purposes. Instincts in humans (and primates) are less fixed and more flexible, take longer to develop, and are more variably expressed than in less complex animals.

In both Jung's theory of archetype and Bowlby's theory of human instinct, typical emotional response patterns arise at certain points in the human life cycle, and concern communications essential to survival needs. These patterns are connected with activities such as infant bonding, peer play, curiosity, hierarchical dominance, initiation rituals, territorial aggression, and the like. Jung said the following of archetype as it relates to instinct in humans:

> Instincts are by no means blind, spontaneous, isolated impulses; they are on the contrary associated with typical situational patterns and cannot be released unless existing conditions correspond to the *a priori* pattern. The collective contents expressed in mythologems represent such situational patterns, which are so intimately connected with the release of instinct. For this reason, knowledge of them is of the highest practical importance to the psychotherapist. (1966, p. 92)

Stevens (1982) has recently argued for the superiority of Jung's concept of archetype over Bowlby's (1969) instinct, in that Jung's idea includes the symbolic expression connected to the typical social instincts of people, the symbolizing animals. States of emotional arousal—fear, attachment, separation—are symbolized in traditional stories and human rituals, as well as expressed individually in gesture and language. The archetype as such is evident in integrated patterns of physiological arousal, in gestural expression, and in typical motifs and themes in the common stories and rituals across cultures. The range of potential human expression of instinctual response, through meaning, is much greater than for other animals. What it *means* to feel angry, loving, or fearful is expressed in many elaborate, though typical, ways by humans.

The concept of archetype permits us to understand what is archaic and enduring in human communication. Archetypes are the organizing cores of meaning for complexes whose specific content must be interpreted with regard to an individual's particular life experience in a particular culture. Complexes are not communicated in rational language. Their meaning is implied, infused with emotion, and larger than life in an ordinary sense. The negative Mother complex, for example, is a collection of qualities, images, feelings, and ideas around the archetypal image of the Terrible Mother, the negative aspect of attachment. When this complex is experienced, through identification or projection, a person feels a serious threat of symbiosis, stagnation, or even death. Jung's psychology assumes that the ego complex, or the experience of "I," is always under threat by unconscious complexes.

Jung's (e.g., 1966) second major contribution to therapeutic practice is his insistence that *unity in the personality is an achievement*. Although he contends that humans are predisposed to strive for unity in personal identity, the experience of a unified self is never automatic or given. Both at any moment and over a life span, the unity of a person—in terms of consciousness, intentionality, and self-consistency—is an achievement. Therefore, we cannot assume that we are speaking with a person who will consistently display a particular set of attitudes and assumptions that is as unified as the physical body appears to be. Rather, a person is made up of different and competing complexes, which are usually resolved into some central experience of "I" (the ego complex) consisting of an image of the physical self and a sense of personal agency in action.

Jung (e.g., 1969b) called the universal striving for coherence the "archetype of Self" and capitalized the word to distinguish it from an individual's experience in a particular life context. Jung's archetype of Self is similar to Winnicott's idea of "continuity of being" (Davis & Wallbridge, 1981); that is, it seems to be the foundation upon which all other human experience is built. From the time personal identity comes into being, through the differentiation of the body and a sense of being and doing, an individual, according to Winnicott, strives for continuity. The success or failure of this striving depends on how securely this person has made attachments with other people and maintains the feeling of being "held" or "contained" in ongoing relationships. Jung does not stress the contribution of attachment to the experience of Self; rather, he stresses the importance of an intrapsychic "container" or framework of meaning that will accommodate both conscious and unconscious strivings toward a coherent personality, as well as emphasizing the importance of living a symbolic life and of establishing a relationship to one's dream images.

Obviously, not every woman achieves a consistent identity. Especially because of our current social conditions, women have a strong propensity to experience themselves as fragmented, often divided between the Mother complex and the animus complex. Our scheme for the growth and integration of the animus complex in women stresses the importance of interpersonal relationships in the development of the *female self*, while from Jung's psychology, we assume that an innate potential for wholeness or integration is supported by the dialectical process of dreaming (dialogue among complexes). Jung's (1969b) idea of compensation, balancing conscious and unconscious thought forms, is especially informative for psychotherapy and is fundamental to our thesis about the development of the animus in women. He credits unconscious thought, as expressed in dreams, nonrational behavior, and symbolic expression, with as much intelligence and meaning as conscious, rational thought.

Gender identity, although only one aspect of personal identity, is central to the way we view ourselves. Because every known society has some scheme that creates social differentiation based on biological difference (Sherif, 1982), we understand gender to be founded on a basic archetype of difference. We think of this as an archetype of opposites, or the instinctive tendency to discriminate between self and not-self. Social categories of gender differences present some typical themes across cultures, but these are not clearly enough established to allow the conclusion that there are specific archetypal differences between women and men. Because the means for establishing gender identity within cultural contexts are varied, any psychological study of women must include their specific social contexts. We have therefore decided against conceptualizing universal archetypes of feminine and masculine, in favor of studying gender themes that are typical in our own society.

Animus, as we have said before, is a psychological complex comprising the excluded aspects of female gender identity: images, ideas, feelings, and action patterns which are associated with the opposite sex. We further hypothesize that the complex is organized by the archetype of the opposite or Not-I, which is reworked around contrasexual elements after gender differentiation has taken place. The essential factor in animus psychology is the relationship between the experiencing subject (girl/woman) and her complex. In an adult woman, animus is experienced as the emotionally charged internal constructs through which she understands and anticipates the world of males and masculine meaning. The actual content of any woman's animus complex depends upon the sorts of influences her social group has had on her, upon what she knows about her own gender identity, upon her perceptions of the opposite sex, and upon the progress of her own personality development.

Animus seems to be the unconscious source for representations of known and unknown men (and "men-animals") in women's dreams. It is also the basis of fantasies about men, their power, and their authority. Because of it, a woman approaches the masculine world with underlying predispositions, assumptions, and affective responses. Because of the particular organization of our society and the greater social influence allowed to men, most adult women have excluded the qualities of personal authority and competence from their conscious gender identity. Only if a woman projects or identifies with the unconscious animus complex, as she is bound to do in her relationships with men, do these qualities become charged by emotions. Then her self-esteem will rise or fall as she begins to regard herself in the way she thinks a man would, that is, from the perspective of her animus.

Jung's (1969b) concept of *individuation,* or the successive integration of unconscious complexes over an entire life span, is the overarching model we use in our approach to psychotherapy. In classical Jungian theory, the integration of the animus complex into conscious self-awareness occurs in middle and later life. After working with women of all ages, however, we have discovered that the process of achieving unity with animus is a prominent element in the therapy of all our adult clients. As they begin to assume responsibility for the qualities they project onto men, male authority figures, and male-dominated institutions (such as the university), women experience a stronger sense of personal authority and self-determination. They also become more able to perceive and accept men as individuals rather than as emotionally charged aspects of their own identities, because they are less dependent on men for validating their personal worth.

The integration of the animus complex is outlined in the accompanying diagram. On the left are the stages of animus development, which are discussed in detail later. The horizontal lines represent the personality of the moment. The portions of any line that fall outside of the funnel shape indicate the strength of the unconscious complex. Inside the funnel shape is the woman's secure sense of self as female.

INTEGRATION OF THE ANIMUS COMPLEX

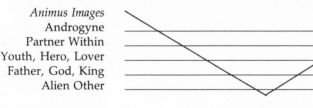

Female Self

As a woman gradually comes to include in her conscious picture of herself more and more of what she had previously excluded as alien to her gender identity, she begins to feel more whole, more completely human, and more androgynous. Naturally, this kind of integration is a struggle, especially in a society that is not supportive, as the case descriptions in Chapters 5–11 will illustrate. In using the therapeutic relationship to assist women, we are guided by Jung's (1966) third major contribution to psychotherapy: *The way humans relate to them-*

selves and others is governed by simultaneously different, competing modes of reality.

In order to work with unconscious complexes in therapy, we interpret human communication from three perspectives, which we derive from Jung's psychology. The first is the perspective of the *archetype as such*. At this level of communication, basic human instinctual–emotional expression takes the form of gesture, posture, and movement (e.g., rocking, falling asleep, holding). The second mode of reality is the *unconscious* (or *archetypal*) *complex*. Complexes are expressed in projections, dream images (usually personified), symbolic or ritualistic actions (e.g., compulsive cleaning), and in moods. They are experienced as alien and emotionally charged states of being, hypersensitivity, and habitual actions. Complexes are interpreted or understood through amplification in systems of symbols such as universal mythologems or motifs from art, literature, and religion. The third perspective for our work is that of *personal identity* (what Jung calls the "ego complex"). Personal identity is expressed as a personal narrative, which is historical and largely rational. Much of the work of therapy focuses on reconstructing the client's personal narrative and exploring it for new meaning. A life story is initially put together out of whatever contextual rules derive from an individual's family of origin and social group. Personal identity is experienced as a center in the self that strives to be autonomous and coherent.

Psychotherapy assists clients in expanding personal identity and in accommodating conflicting experiences and ideas within a unified narrative. This is all part of the work of integrating the animus complex with the conscious self. The purpose of this chapter has been to clarify the underlying assumptions and theoretical concepts we bring to our analysis of female authority. Although we will use other theoretical systems in developing our topic further, here we have attempted to present our framework for discussing competence, feminism, and Jung's psychology.

4

The Animus and I:
A Model for Psychotherapy
with Women

In mothering, caregiving, and related activities, women are assumed to be emotionally powerful. Among adults, however, a woman's insistence on her personal convictions is frequently denigrated and carries little social impact. The direct authority of an adult woman often has a paradoxical effect on other adults: It is both emotionally powerful and ineffectual.

Many of us were mothered by women who suffered from low self-esteem, who were socially confined to household and immediate family, and who have been called "self-less." In adulthood, we may have a confusing sense that Mother was (and perhaps is) both powerful and inferior. We may imagine that she was domineering, contemptuous, weak, or manipulative. Given our social conditioning, it is unlikely that we believe her mothering was ideal or even well suited to our needs. This woman's forceful will and emotional expressiveness were uniquely motivating for us during a phase of our lives when we were vulnerable and thus vitally dependent on her. Not only were we small and contained within her care, but we did not have available rational or reflective thought—or even a language—by which to conceive of this female power.

In adult life, then, most of us are ambivalent about female authority, especially an insistent and emotional authority. Experiencing a woman's aggression, anger, persuasion, or fear connects us to nonrational experiences and influences that may still seem threatening, overwhelming, and in opposition to our own will or impulses.

NEGATIVE MOTHER COMPLEX AND ANIMUS COLLUSION

Three psychosocial conditions appear to contribute to the devaluation of female nurturing and the fear of women's authority. The first one has already been discussed in previous chapters: the presumed inferiority of female gender (i.e., that women are less competent, less intelligent, etc., than men). The other two are analyzed here as the basis for understanding the effects of the "negative Mother complex" on contemporary women who are attempting to claim their own authority.

The second condition is the paradoxical nature of female emotional power. The voice of female insistence is stereotypically characterized as attacking the freedom of men to be independent and rational, in both family and work settings. Women's anger, aggression and fear are pejoratively described as engulfing and overwhelming, impossible for men to understand or manage. Chodorow (1978) and Dinnerstein (1976) offer helpful analyses about how this situation has evolved. By opposing feminine traits and refusing female authority, a boy forms an independent identity from the powerful female of his infancy and childhood. He develops his identity (typically) with few readily available male role models. In this kind of environment, his emotional investment tends more toward opposing the female, both within and outside of himself, rather than emulating the male. The little boy does not simply separate and individuate from his mother. He actively opposes and represses her effects on his identity. This aspect of male socialization is readily in evidence, but one obvious example will carry the point: There is no social context in which a little boy can be proud to be a "sissy," like a little girl can be proud to be a "tomboy."

The paradoxical power of female mothering creates identity defenses in men especially, whereby they are prone to resist female authority and to oppose its emotional force. Forceful directives from women in adult relationships are often labeled by men in ways that inhibit a woman's self-esteem: as bitchy, castrating, and the like. These labels, while they imply an interpersonal power, are confusing because they do not mean that a woman is having a dominant social influence on the man who uses them. For instance, a woman may be called "domineering" by her husband at the very moment he adamantly refuses to follow her directive (even a simple "Close the door.").

The paradox of female power has consequences among women as well. Although a woman may not be inhibited or overwhelmed by an insistent or angry statement made by another woman, she may become so uncomfortable that she disregards the content. Because she also has individuated from a woman, she has defenses against powerful female authority and she has internalized some assumptions about the inferiority of her gender. Without consciously opposing her own defense against female authority, an adult woman will also tend to receive female power reluctantly and to seek male validation for her convictions.

The third major psychosocial condition that contributes to the devaluing and fear of female authority is the separation of men from women and their work, especially in areas of personal style and nurturing. In most adult settings of American society, a grown man in a dress and wearing makeup would be thought "odd," although women wear men's pants and ties without disapproval. Men must exclude the feminine from their identity far more vigilantly and strenuously than women have to exclude the masculine. Men feel compelled to "fight the feminine" unless they are identified with being homosexual, members of a sexual-perference group that shares with women some of the social stigma of being feminine.

Large-scale studies (e.g., as cited in Eagly, 1983) of time spent by men and women on child care and housework continue to reveal evidence that men separate themselves from women's work. Similarly, in social settings outside the home, men are represented as small minorities in secretarial, nursing, social work, elementary school teaching, and nursery care professions.

Because men hold powerful decision-making positions, control material resources, and are rewarded with other symbols of authority, their distance from the world of female power (nurturance and emotional life) is an implicit message that the dominant members of our society may experience our power as negative or inferior. Whereas they idealize the institution of motherhood in terms of emotional virtue, they do not reward its activities with symbolic indicators of authority. On a daily basis, it is clear that the "men in charge" do not compete for primary roles of nurturing, providing care, or sustaining human relationships.

Our broad cultural undervaluing of these roles carries over into women's difficulties in claiming their own authority. Irrational negative responses to forceful female authority, and repression of the worthy aspects of caregiving, are part of a collective psychological problem with mothering: the negative Mother complex, in Jungian terms. Recall that a complex is a collection of ideas, feelings, and actions gathered around a core of emotional arousal. The predisposition to form an image in this aroused state is called an *archetype*, as discussed in the previous chapter. The archetype of Mother is the universal tendency to form an emotionally aroused image of a powerful caregiver upon whom one is entirely dependent in infancy, somewhat dependent in childhood, and from whom one is independent in adulthood. Although the image may result from accumulated care received from many persons and under various conditions, the infant forms a single image of Mother, which is later translated into an internally motivating psychological complex. This complex is then projected onto the woman who has carried the primary care responsibilities of the developing child.

Two poles of expression of the archetype of Mother depict the extremes of emotional power associated with mothering: Great Mother (nurturance, sustenance, enhancement of life, protection) and Terrible Mother (stasis, suffocation, engulfment, death). These archetypal potentials are elements of the human psyche that form in response to typical human dependence in infancy and childhood. They are not personal characteristics of an individual woman. Emotional responses from complexes are always "bigger than life" and beyond the realm of personal responsibility. They connect us to nonrational, symbolic realms of instinctual meaning and to our dependence on other members of the species for survival.

Androcentric norms and assumptions tend to exclude or repress the Great Mother pole of this archetype, having profound effects on our attitudes toward the natural environment, human emotional bonds, and our own bodies. In adulthood we respond to both female power and our own mothers in terms of the Terrible Mother aspect of the archetype. The combination of inferior gender identity with exclusively female mothering results in our devaluing women's power and economically, socially, and politically oppressing the people who emulate the feminine in providing care and nurturance. An emotionally insistent woman who attempts to impose her will or self-interests on other adults can easily become the target of the negative Mother projections in the family, in work settings, and within her own identity.

Let us look at two examples. The first one is a public lecture given by a woman social worker who is talking about her research on father–daughter relationships. She speaks insistently and forcefully about her findings and illustrates her talk with many impressive data. Whether or not her data are convincing and her talk is well presented, she is likely to be evaluated according to identity characteristics of the negative Mother. She may be called overly emotional, overly intellectual, or too pushy, but it is unlikely that her presentation will be assessed solely on its merits.

The second example is an anecdote from Stiver (1983) which is a perfect illustration of how the negative Mother complex is projected in interpersonal relations between women and men. The speaker is Stiver, a woman.

> Recently I was talking to a male colleague about something I considered to be extremely important. I needed his support, and I was talking with a good deal of feeling. He minimized what I said and downplayed its importance . I couldn't agree, and I was getting more and more exasperated. He kept saying, "Well, it's not really that important," or "Let's wait and see." Finally, in a kind of apathetic way, I said quietly, "Well, there's this, this, and that . . . ," enumerating the points again, but this time without any feeling. He said, "Oh, why didn't you say that before—instead of coming on like a witch on a broom." At first I was hurt, then I thought further—I tried to tell him something and let him know it was important, but he couldn't hear me. My intense expression of feeling made him too anx-

ious to hear the message, yet I felt my feelings were just as important to the communication as the words! (pp. 4–5)

In analyzing the anecdote, Stiver stresses the idea that women are made
to feel they must express their ideas without feelings and that they
should detach themselves from their experiences. We would take the
analysis one step further and say that women are pressured to communicate with emotional distance because we all find enactments of
the negative Mother complex deeply uncomfortable. In other words, as
a culture we prefer that women restrict their emotional convictions and
forcefulness because we tend to find them irrationally overwhelming.

When Jung (1959) conceived of the concept of animus, it seems he
meant it to represent primarily an unconscious compensation in women
for a lack of intellectual objectivity.[1] He described a syndrome of attitude
and affect that was shaped around a dogmatic and argumentative
defense of empty opinions. No doubt this formulation of a woman's
inferiority has its roots in the sociocultural context in which Jung made
his initial observations, but it is notable that Jung featured this syndrome as a central problem in women's personalities when *both* men
and women can argue excitedly from empty opinions, and must surely have done so in Swiss society of Jung's day. Perhaps Jung also was
vulnerable to dismissing the validity of the *content* of a woman's explanation when she argued in an excited or anxious manner.

The man in the Stiver quote accuses the woman of "coming on
like a witch on a broom," although she was in fact offering a perspective which he eventually saw as reasonable and valid. The male colleague rejected the rational meaning of Stiver's words when he felt
overwhelmed by the complex. He then accepted their meaning because
he realized she was not, apparently, going to be forceful or insistent.
Because she was a woman, he assumed that she made the interchange
confusing by her emotional insistence. Although the communication
difficulty was apparently in the man's ability to listen, he attributed the
problem to the woman speaker.

The distress of excluded authority in women is neither solely the
result of identifying with negative Mother projections nor of identifying with inferior qualities of female gender. Rather we find a collusion
between the two, in which social and psychological conditions inter-
face to form a powerful force in a woman's development. When a
woman speaks with emotional conviction she is likely to meet with
some negative identity attributions. She will get the attributions whether or not she has something valid to say. She is vulnerable to internalizing negative judgments, especially from male authorities, in regard to

1. See Young-Eisendrath (1984, pp. 23–24) for a fuller discussion of this.

her competence, objectivity, intelligence, etc. While she may be able to resist the negative labeling of her emotional power (e.g., that she is overly demanding), she is less likely able to resist the implications about her thinking or competence. Because she feels certain that the standards for truth, goodness, and beauty rest outside of herself, she is vulnerable to internalizing negative challenges by powerful males and other authority figures. Such challenges are most likely rooted in emotional resistance to a repressed Mother complex.

A woman speaking with a man in authority, or competing for a position in a male-dominated context, is likely to anticipate her performance anxiously although she may be quite competent and well prepared. If she reflects on herself from the perspective of her animus, the anxiety caused by her lowered self-esteem will increase her emotional expressiveness, making her vulnerable both to the interpersonal resistance of men and to a transitory identification with the negative Mother complex in which she experiences her emotionality as "bad" or overwhelming.

As a result of the collusion of the negative Mother and animus complexes in female development, many adult women do not know how to discriminate their own valid authority for making a claim to truth. That is, they readily become confused about whether or not they know something, especially in the presence of men and sometimes of all adults. To put this another way, they have not learned to discriminate between the validity of their own sources and male reflections of their validity.

DEVELOPMENT OF ANIMUS

A woman's capacity to understand her animus complex and to establish a relationship with it evolves developmentally. Certain themes appear at the first emergence of a woman's gender identity and take on other characteristics later. The little girl seeks validation of her power through masculine approval of her appearance or achievements after she separates from her identification with Mother. Necessarily, her self-esteem becomes overly focused on her relationships with men and male standards because they are perceived as powerful and true. Approval and encouragement by her father contributes to a benign or positive animus complex as the girl develops. Lack of involvement with the father, severe or judgmental fathering, and above all, abuse contribute to a negative animus complex. Girls adapt to negative animus either by compensating and appearing to succeed, while internally always falling short (commonly known as "perfectionism"), or by giving up a sense of self-worth and seeking to soothe the anxiety of self-hatred by becoming subservient to men. One way or another, every woman eventually faces identity problems due to the inferiority of female gender. Even when she has a positive animus from childhood, a woman must face men who are not like her father and will not reward and reinforce those qualities her father so adored. Therefore, most women behave in adulthood as though they have to seek power and authority either by becoming like men or by becoming liked by men. We have not met a single woman who has not in some way judged her self-worth by whether or not she was meeting masculine standards.

As we have witnessed the animus developing in women in therapy, it evolves through different images. Individual women enter therapy at different points along the continuum of stages. The first stage is the complex as "alien" or "outsider"—masculinity which is threatening and frightening. The second configuration is a fatherly or god kind of complex, and the third is a lover or heroic complex. Our therapeutic goal in these first three stages is to assist a woman in shifting her attitude from one of approval seeking to one of validating her own authority as a female. To move from the first to the second stage, however, a woman must experience some kind of significant approval in the masculine domain.

Male approval may come via relationships (e.g., with father, brother, or teacher), via work or creative expression (as rewarded in the patriarchy by status or money), via the power of wealth (her own or her spouse's), via beauty or appearance (through male recognition), or any combination of these. Naturally some forms of approval in the masculine domain (e.g., earning an independent income) can be assisted or facilitated through therapy, whereas others (e.g., getting dates) cannot. Because acceptance by the patriarchal world (beyond the household *per se*), either through her own status or through male reflections, contributes to a woman's sense of power, we will assist a woman in the first stage in attaining it. To move beyond the godly or fatherly animus complex (once such masucline approval has been achieved) will mean the conversion of approval into competence, the recognition of herself as "worth it" or as a potential equal with men.

At later stages (Stages Four and Five) of animus development, in which the woman experiences herself as having a "good-enough" man within, the woman becomes freer to function as a whole person. Essentially, she will have expanded her gender identity to include many of the behaviors and attributions formerly excluded as male or masculine. She feels free to behave and validate herself in a wide range of activities, without excessive anxiety or approval seeking. Such a woman is less likely to develop identity relationships with men or with her children. She experiences herself as legitimate in her own right with the skill and competence of her work incorporated into her self-concept. At these later stages, women feel free to enjoy themselves among other woman in a new way. They are no longer so completely focused on power concerns or competition "among inferiors." In other words, they are no longer prone to identify with the negative Mother complex.

That women typically adapt to the inferior status accorded to their authority is a larger cultural concern, and from our perspective, involvement in some aspect of the women's movement is the only effective way to reclaim the legitimacy of one's identity as a worthwhile human being. In other words, the way to focus development of the animus complex for a particular woman is to empower her. A woman, by experiencing competence, gradually learns not to internalize the deficits that are projected onto her gender. While this process of development includes "consciousness raising" and concern for the broader social issues, the psychological components of assisting women in developing a benign and positive animus complex also involve reworking the effects of relationships to men and male institutions.

Certainly not all of our clients arrive at the final stages of development conceptualized here. Past and present life circumstances can prevent a complete development of the animus complex and a complete reworking of unconscious tendencies to experience female gender identity as inferior. Many clients, however, are able to achieve a better relationship to the animus and to increase self-esteem and personal authority in the course of therapy. Our hope is to move with our clients closer to a state of being in which they become freer to commit themselves to their ideals and work, to relate to both men and women openly, and to resist negative attributions about both.

Psychotherapists who aim to empower women as individuals must themselves work for social changes. If they do not, individual therapy takes on a pall of hopelessness and depression. Depression is an ongoing problem for all of us as we recognize to what degree women are truly the victims of male dominance and greed. Women are also the easiest targets for blame, especially since they are mothers. Similarly, they are targets of impossible wishes, especially for a "completely responsive Other." This is not to say that men are to blame. We all participate in the patriarchy, and we are all responsible for it. Empowering women and making a cultural decision to value caregiving and the ordinary tasks of life will free us to cooperate more fully and with greater emotional reward in interpersonal relationships.

None of what we say here or elsewhere about the animus complex and the inferior authority of women is intended to diminish the concerns or belittle the competence of mothering. On the contrary, we recognize that mothering is one of the most rewarding and necessary of human activities, and believe that if we are to revitalize ourselves as women, we cannot continue to regard mothering as a low-status activity. Instead we recognize the skill and complexity of mothering in general, and then go one step further. Revaluing self-worth and ac- tualizing dependence as a female ultimately include *embracing one's own mother*. To embrace one's mother is to free her of the negative Mother complex and to see her realistically as an individual in a particular life context.

At later stages of animus development, revaluing the mother's role leads to new respect for her skills. We no longer denigrate the ability to care for others by assuming that it involves no intelligence or training. Responding to complex interpersonal cues, understanding nonrational communication, and managing the activities of a family are appreciated as responsible and intelligent activities. Validation of mothering skills should also extend to the caregiving professions, which at present are socially oppressed in our society.

A MODEL FOR GIRLS AND WOMEN: EGO DEVELOPMENT AND ANIMUS DEVELOPMENT

In social and psychological functioning, the female sense of self must be conceived in *both* interpersonal and intrapsychic terms. Jungian psychologists have tended to emphasize an intrapsychic model and to deemphasize or exclude the interpersonal dimension of relationships in personality formation. Female identity in our society evolves through significant relationships, first from an "identity relationship" between at least two females. Contributing to the girl's gender identity are two conditions: identification with a powerful person of the same gender and exclusion of certain personal characteristics as male, to be projected onto the opposite gender. Let us again emphasize that in tracing the development of identity in girls and women, we need to keep in mind both what is consciously accepted as part of the female self-concept and what is consciously or unconsciously excluded.

To supplement the intrapsychic model of Jung's psychology, we have chosen Loevinger's (1976) ego development model to map the dif- ferentiation of a female self-concept within relationship and society. We find this model useful for clinical assessments of self–other meaning in the context of both competence and vulnerability. Moreover, the logic of ego development, from Loevinger's research, has guided our obser- vations of animus development and provided a conceptual scheme for the sequencing of animus images we have encountered in our clinical work.

Despite its title, Loevinger's model is not focused on ego autonomy, or an unconflicted ego sphere, as the outcome of healthy development. Taking her initial orientation from the interpersonal psychology of

Sullivan (1953), Loevinger has evolved a model that accounts for the development of self in relation to other. For our purposes, her model has several features that make it preferable to others. First and foremost, it was devised from and validated through research on thousands of girls and woman. Using a sentence completion test, Loevinger collected data from females over a 25-year period while she gradually filled out a system of nine stages from an initial outline of four developmental positions reasoned from Sullivan's theory.

Loevinger's first major contribution to ego development theory bore the earmarks of her extensive training and earlier research in psychometrics. The first two volumes on ego development (Loevinger & Wessler, 1970) are instruction and scoring manuals for the sentence completion test she uses. These manuals serve as the best introduction to the intricacies of development in her scheme, which combines interpersonal, cognitive, and moral functions. The manuals contain hundreds of actual completions, organized by exemplary categories, of 36 incomplete sentences such as "A pregnant woman. . . . " Sentence completions provide insight into broad and specific characteristics of female development from the earliest differentiation of impulses to the final achievements of self-actualization.

Loevinger's second major contribution to personality theory is her theoretical work *Ego Development* (1976), which gives a complete account of the history and synthesis of her conceptual scheme. Although she refuses to define the concept of ego in a tightly constraining way, Loevinger clearly articulates the assumptions underlying her constructs. Ego means the more or less systematic way in which an individual brings coherence to the experience of self and world. (The predisposition to formulate an ego attitude, or to strive for coherence, is what Jung means by the archetype of Self.) On a moment-to-moment basis, ego is a synthetic process of bringing to bear a frame of reference for constructing self-and-other concepts. Each of Loevinger's stages presents a paradigm from which a person derives habitual assumptions, hypotheses, and other patterns of action and thought.

Loevinger's (1976) model of development is derived entirely from empirical research using her sentence completion test. Our model resonates with her findings, but it is the product of clinical observations and intuitive common sense. Loevinger has differentiated nine stages, while we have defined only five thematic clusterings of animus complexes. Our observations have been collected through thousands of hours of therapeutic work with women clients, much of it analytical in nature. Most of our therapeutic clients are characterized by the features of the first three stages of animus development, with the majority at the first two. Large-scale research on women's dreams and fantasies would probably result in more differentiated animus stages than offered here.

Ego development stages and self-animus themes fall along a continuum from least to most differentiated, from external to internal cues, and from reactive to proactive. Each new stage provides a fresh framework of meaning that incorporates what has come before in a new, more complex and more integrated structure. In this review of ego and animus development, we emphasize two areas of personality functioning: personal authority and objective empathy. Loevinger does not have a particular theory of either, although she comments on the emergence of true empathy as a rather late developmental achievement. We have imposed our orientation on her scheme and take full responsibility for any errors in our interpertation of her work.

Empathy is the ability to infer another's frame of reference. We add the adjective "objective" in order to stress the accuracy with which the individual strives to see and to separate that frame of reference from her own subjectivity or desire. Through *objective empathy* one is able to feel the emotions of others and to infer the implicit meaning of their communications, both verbal and nonverbal. Objective empathy is possible only after an individual has adequately experienced fusion, attachment, projection, conformity, and sympathy with a variety of others. Empathy integrates all of these other states of being and adds to them the subject's desire for objective accuracy in understanding another.

Authority, as defined earlier, is the power to claim for one's self truth, beauty, or worth. Personal authority is achieved only after an individual has learned to distinguish impulse from control, to understand the consequences of interpersonal actions, to anticipate consequences, to know when one is materially and emotionally dependent, and to take responsibility for one's own thoughts and feelings. To personal authority we add the dimension of "personal limitation," or the idea that responsibility is personally limited in one's life context by depth of commitment and breadth of knowledge. No person has final authority outside of a context.

Ego development, while it represents a continuum from childhood to adulthood, can also be considered a typology of differences among adults. Holt (1980) conducted a national survey of young adults, carefully sampled to represent a broad cross-section of the American population, and verified what Loevinger had deduced from her research on college students: that young adults seem to stop developing at Loevinger's Self-Aware Stage, just beyond conformity. At least until the age of 25, most adults remain at the Self-Aware Stage and adapt to their life contexts out of that stage. Development beyond this stage may be anxiety provoking and stressful because it is not supported by the majority and may isolate individuals from consensual validation of peers and family members.

Loevinger's (1976) ego stages can be seen as ideal types of adult

functioning, whereas the animus complexes should be viewed as clusterings of affectively charged schemata for relating to men and masculine ideals and institutions. Loevinger's research has necessarily
resulted in a focus on what an individual can produce in a conscious
(written) form in response to vague cues (sentence stems). Our clinical
concern has been to systematize what is produced in projections, nonrational communication, dreams, and anticipations. The following summaries are titled by Loevinger's ego development stages. The typical
accompanying animus complex is reviewed briefly as a part of the ego
development stage.

Presocial Stage

When an adult is functioning at the Presocial Stage, she is severely
distressed, dissociated, regressed, delusional, or retarded. The pre-
dominant modes of self–other relating are gestural and kinesthetic. The
form of interactive relationship with others is symbiotic fusion, and
there is no reliable linguistic communication of shared symbolic meaning. Confusing concrete reality with emotional states, projective identification, and other forms of misidentifying self as other, predominate
in interpersonal relationships. Symbiotic fusion with the mothering-
one constitutes the major interpersonal form of relatedness at this stage.
Whether she is in early life or in later adulthood, a person at this stage
is not responsible for her actions, cannot anticipate her needs regularly, and must be provided a protected environment in order to develop
further (in adulthood this usually takes the form of institutionalization).
Unconscious complexes dominate the interpersonal field, and the individual displays herself in terms of highly idiosyncratic expressions
such as shifting moods, hallucinatory states, and gestures and motions
like sucking, rocking, and grasping.

The stage of animus development which is implicit and not consciously recognized is that of animus as Alien Outsider. This alien
character of the complex is undifferentiated but is clearly outside of the
Mother–Daughter symbiotic fusion. The therapeutic relationship with
an adult female client at this stage involves appropriate custodial care
and primary differentiation of self and other. Nonlinguistic therapy
(e.g., movement and art therapy) is the treatment of choice, accompanied by constant reinforcement of "you" and "I" boundaries.

In healthy chronological development, this stage depicts the symbiotic fusion of infant–parent that occurs roughly from conception until some time between 3 and 9 months when differentiation between
self and other emerges in the infant as "stranger anxiety." The first
reliable social smiling done by the infant is a signal that the Presocial

Stage is coming to an end. Social signals that can be interpreted reliably arise in relationship to a separate other.

Impulsive Stage

Self in the Impulsive Stage is experienced as actions and gestures, which are claimed as "I," "me," and "mine." Impulses, habitual behaviors, and patterns of action are more prominent than verbal communications. Ritualistic actions, needs, and feelings are experienced primarily in bodily states of arousal. Feelings in adulthood are described in vague and impoverished ways, such as being "upset," "okay," or "out of it." Needs are experienced as insatiable and dominating so that a woman may fear her own needs as though they were going to destroy her. Unconscious complexes dominate the interactive field and personal control of them seems impossible. Addiction to drugs or alcohol, and difficulties with eating (such as severe binging) express this person's ravaging needs. Addictive preoccupations (e.g., eating or drug abuse) can cause a woman to regress to this stage and operate primarily out of an impulsive orientation, even after she has reached a further stage of ego development.

Ambivalence is the most obvious mode of interpersonal relationship and is often acted out in ways that are confusing to others. For example, clinging dependence may be accompanied by frequent distancing rages. Expressed meanings will tend to dichotomize people and events into "good to me" and "mean to me." Motivation for further development involves immediate need gratification. Support and reinforcement have not been internalized.

The woman assumes that some "authority" controls resources in an arbitrary way. She cannot perceive even the immediate consequences of her interpersonal actions, so she does not distinguish between cause and effect in relating to others. Unconsciously, the woman learns through reward and punishment, and will severely punish herself and others when something goes wrong.

In therapy, this kind of woman conveys a feeling of insatiable hunger. Intimate others are viewed as sources of protection and gratification. The therapeutic relationship involves protective guidance and the teaching of delayed gratification and basic social skills. Behavioral reinforcement of this learning is especially effective. Verbal interpretations should focus on the difference between feelings and actions.

The animus complex continues to be Alien Outsider, but here the masculine Other may in fact be a rapist or abuser. The potential for violent acts between women and men is very high at the Impulsive Stage. Wife abuse, rape, and child abuse are common problems when actions are impulsive and feelings are unarticulated.

The chronological period of healthy development that is depicted here is the time between about 9 months and 3 years of age. At this period, the separation and differentiation of infant and parent creates an interactive field animated by control, opposing emotional pulls, and ambivalence.

Self-Protective Stage

Experiences of individual agency ("I do") and subjectivity ("I, me, mine") are clearly differentiated at the Self-Protective Stage. Struggles of will with others and oppositional attitudes about protecting her own territory are outgrowths of a woman's new development in knowing her self-interest. Preoccupations with interpersonal advantage and control are prominent in relationships. These preoccupations may be observed to be "opportunistic" by others; they seem to be motivated by fears of being overwhelmed by her own needs or alternately of being invaded by others' demands.

A woman at this stage can anticipate the concrete consequences of her actions, a cognitive achievement over the Impulsive Stage. Although she has foresight about the rewards or punishments connected to her actions, she cannot analyze her behavior; she does not understand or recognize her motivations or desires as they arise. Stereotyping and dualistic thinking are common, especially regarding issues of social power (e.g., treating a subordinate very differently from a superior).

Maintaining a hedonistic attitude about her daily life, a woman at this stage will seek immediate gratifications and pleasures, and will avoid pain. Whatever she interprets as work or effort (from personal chores to earning a living) will be viewed primarily as a burden or trouble. Her moral reasoning tends to be concrete: Being wrong *is* getting caught or punished. This kind of concrete hedonism can result in drug, food, and/or alcohol abuse, especially when a woman is stressed or anxious.

In therapy this client will manipulate the therapist in order to gratify herself. She does not feel guilty in doing so, although she may seem ashamed. Because she believes that "an eye for an eye, and a tooth for a tooth" is the ethic for all interpersonal relating, she assumes that the therapist has the same standards as herself. The client is convinced that the therapist will manipulate her for the therapist's own ends (e.g., making money), and the client will attempt to do the same. "Everyone is out to get a free lunch" is the social motto for this stage. The client will project her feelings of hostility and aggression onto the therapist. She will not feel conflicts in herself over these feelings. The animus complex can be projected onto men or women, and the therapist can become the target for the complex even at the beginning of therapy.

In the therapeutic relationship, benefits of interpersonal trust and conformity should be stressed. Concrete pleasure (e.g., "soothing") can be used to reinforce this learning. The sense of structure and the reliability and the concern of the therapist form the context for further development. Management of the therapeutic session by an expert and unshakable therapist becomes essential in the face of hostility, ambivalence, accusation, and acting out of impulses.

The animus complex continues to be largely Alien Outsider, although one may see the beginnings of the patriarchal complex of Father, God, or King. The complex is usually negative and punishing although it may be idealized and projected as an absolute authority, such as a male god. In such a case, the woman will attempt to fashion herself according to the directives of this god in order to attain personal rewards for herself. Relationships with men are intensely ambivalent and unreliable, and they emphasize material dependence.

The chronological period comparable to this stage is that time from roughly 3 years to 6 years of age in healthy development. Children develop the "magic" of lying during this time and learn to manipulate reality to their own ends. Opportunistic bending of rules in children's games, struggles for dominance, and escape into power fantasies are normal preoccupations in interpersonal functioning.

Conformist Stage

Belonging to a group and being identified with it are the benchmarks for achieving a conformist orientation. In adulthood, women at the Conformist Stage usually consider their family of origin as their primary point of reference. They strive for approval and acceptance, and especially seek to conform to the dictates of authority within their reference groups. Standards for appearance, behavior, and preferences preoccupy their thinking. Self-esteem is engendered through acceptance and approval by her group rather than through simple hedonistic rewards.

Meeting the needs of others is a major avenue to acceptance. Needs are conceptualized in stereotypical ways, which confuse individual and group differences. Dualistic judgments of "right–wrong" and "good–bad" result in a rather simplistic categorization of people. Old people, teenagers, and ethnic and racial groups are viewed in terms of stereotypes, which usually derive from the woman's family of origin. A woman at this stage might explain, for instance, that her teenage son is "rowdy because all teenagers are rowdy." Niceness and helpfulness are directed toward the groups that define her self-concept. Prejudice and fear are directed toward outsiders, who are broadly considered to be "stupid" or "weird." When such a woman breaks with the standards of her group, she becomes very anxious about her social status. Severe stress in her self-concept may emerge around a concern as simple as serving the "wrong" food for a holiday celebration.

Traditional female gender identity is congruent with the ideals of conformity. Dependency, submissiveness to authority, niceness, and a need to belong are features of both. A woman may identify her self-concept with conformity throughout her adult life without being considered maladjusted or inadequate from a social perspective. Psychologically, however, she will experience severe anxiety and depression over questions regarding her ability to be an active personal agent in her own life. She will defend against these feelings, at least in part, by attributing immorality or ignorance to "outsiders."

The animus complex usually has the form of Alien Outsider when the woman overidentifies with her family of origin and the traditions of Mother within it. Through a strong unconscious identity with matriarchal power, the woman experiences the male as alien. The animus complex can also take the form of Father, God, or King and become the dominant authority for the woman's actions. The husband, father, male god, or male political leader is viewed as intrinsically powerful and legitimate in his authority when the complex is shaped by the power of the patriarch.

In the therapeutic relationship, we see the first signs of true personal authority and objective empathy emerging in interpersonal relating. The woman begins to use other people as reference points rather than material support. When she imitates the leaders of her group, she will confront the problem of self-assertion. She will begin to note the reality of different frames of reference as she seeks to belong to different reference groups (e.g., at church and in the neighborhood). Although her niceness and helpfulness are more conforming than sympathetic or empathic, they involve her in feeling others' experience. "Feeling sorry for" and "being upset about" others' pain and stress are the first signs of developing empathy. Similarly, the woman's growing awareness of the power of appearance may engender an understanding of self-control different from her earlier ideas of manipulation. A client will be alert to her therapist's appearance and pain. She will want the therapist to look good and feel good, and she will feel sorry if these conditions are not manifest. Consistent and reliable support from the therapist in teaching clarification of values and decision making, as well as using different words for states of feeling, is conducive to the woman's further development. Group therapy can be especially useful in helping the woman learn to differentiate between her own feelings and preferences and those of other individuals.

The chronological period which roughly corresponds to conformity is the time between 7 years and 18 or 19 years of age. This is an extended period of time when the girl identifies herself with peer groups if she is confident in moving out of her family of origin. At the beginning of this period, the young girl cannot distinguish between appearances and feelings. She confuses "pretty" with "nice," and she elaborates her interpersonal awareness by distinguishing among different types of appearance. Near the end of the conformist period, she should have achieved adequate interpersonal modes of attachment-separation, dominance–submission, and dependence–independence within her peer group. Her relationship to boys and men, especially to her own father, will contribute importantly to her ability to accept differences in herself and others.

Self-Aware Stage

Up to this stage, self-concept and self-esteem have been attached primarily to imitation and approval of others. Until now, identity relationships with parents, peers, siblings, and teachers have formed the bases for a woman's ideals and values.

At the Self-Aware Stage, a woman is awakened (either gradually or suddenly) to a recognition of diversity in norms and values as legitimate. Although her thinking style will continue to be somewhat stereotyping and dualistic, she will become aware that legitimate differences of values and moral standards exist among different people. She will, however, tend to assume these differences are inherent in "the way people are" (or a similar cliché) rather than seeing how they are connected to cultural or knowledge systems. Consequently, she may accept differences in beliefs or moral standards as legitimate for diverse groups (e.g., different standards for Jews and Christians), but she will not be able to reason about these differences in regard to their origins in particular contexts. She will not be able to assume different points of view confidently although she knows they exist in the world.

Belonging and approval are still the primary motives for increases in self-esteem, but a woman will struggle with her personal authority over her own independence. Paradoxically, she seeks the approval of an authority to validate her difference. She wants someone in authority to tell her repeatedly that her independence is "good." Conflicting roles are the arena for further development. Imposing an ideal of self-consistency in enacting the roles of dependent wife, authoritative mother, and confident expert will increase the woman's anxiety about her self-concept. She cannot reconcile differences within her own needs and desires in different reference groups because she has bound her self-esteem to the approval of authority, usually male.

Motivated by a conscious desire to be rational and logical (since these are male ideals), the woman wishes to plan for the future and to articulate her own life goals in a "sensible" way. The conscious idea of a goal as the "key to success" emerges spontaneously at this stage. Talking about personal goals and feelings can be rewarding in and of itself. The desire to become conscious of self as an individual is usually experienced within these kinds of conversations as an exciting potential. (An older woman may be intensely afraid to ask the question "Who am I?" because she fears that nobody but herself cares about the answer. She may also fear that she has lost the opportunity to discover the answer and to make use of it in her life.)

Because personal meanings are perceived in more complex ways than in earlier stages, a woman in this stage may actually be frightened by the multiplicity of norms and standards in human life. Confused by her new ideal that "everyone has a right to an opinion," the woman begins to feel lost in a sea of limitless possibilities. Right–wrong, good–bad, and self–other are no longer discrete and reliable internal categories. Because she has no coherently established self-concept, and because she has externalized authority and internalized inferiority, the woman feels acute pressure about her desire to find herself. Although she may not verbally state her anxiety about old standards of appearance and values, she will appear pressured when making decisions about changing her life-style, her orientation, and her appearance. Such a woman is vulnerable to acute anxiety and depression over these issues. Feeling a lack of control over what previously seemed determined by others, and suffering from unpredictable anxiety about self-esteem, this woman may repeatedly give herself over to unconscious complexes, which leave her helpless rather than strengthened by a legitimate personal point of view.

In some ways, the therapeutic relationship is more difficult at this stage than at previous ones. The extremes of ambivalence were enacted in the dependence and rage of earlier ego development stages, but now the woman becomes more consciously skeptical about female authority—both her own and the therapist's (if female). The client is suspicious of identifying authority with femaleness, and she will test the therapist's expertise and validity in a way reminiscent of an adolescent daughter testing the advice of her mother. The client will feel that she knows more about life and male–female struggles than the therapist does. Although such a woman may be sympathetic to the women's movement, she will project her own feelings of inferiority and aggression onto other women. She finds it especially difficult to believe in female authority figures, may fight the therapist, and frequently resists change in a variety of inventive conscious and unconscious ways.

The typical form of the animus complex is patriarchal. We find some retreat to animus as Alien Outsider in both younger and older women. A preoccupation with male–female power struggles can lead to distrust of males. Equality based on mutuality and reciprocity is not consciously understood but becomes an ideal. The value of equal partnership with men can be used to reinforce the work of therapy. Teaching women values-clarification, decision-making, and social skills for independent living is an important aspect of therapy. Supportive clarification of strengths and competences, and role modeling provide the right interpersonal environment for building trust of female authority.

The chronological period that corresponds to the Self-Aware Stage is early adulthood, roughly from 19 to 28 years of age. This is the classic time for men to resolve the "identity crisis" of their developing self-concept. For women, this is the classic time to defer their own identity crisis by forming an "identity relationship" with a man. Young women are vulnerable to "loss of self" when they form intense identity relationships with men at this period. If they marry the person onto whom they have projected the patriarchal animus complex, they are at risk for continuing their identification of self-worth with the partner. The partner's achievements, independence, and knowledge replace the woman's own need for development. Because of her adaptation to the roles of wife and mother, the woman is at risk for severe depression in middle or later life.

Conscientious Stage

For the first time, there clearly emerges a conscious awareness of a past and future that relates to the present. In the Conscientious Stage a woman can see patterns in her own development and may actually discover the idea of psychological development spontaneously. Personal achievement and responsibility are the affectively charged themes of interpersonal relating at this stage. Desires for achievement and a feeling of responsibility for others provoke a true identity crisis in which the woman articulates the question "Who am I?"

Because conceptual complexity, complete formal thought operations, and some sense of personal identity have been achieved, a woman can relate empathically. She has a full repertoire of emotional responses and words to express them. Mutuality and cooperation are conscious ideals and are rooted in concern for the welfare of others. Guilt may become a prominent feeling in the woman's life because she will tend to take too much responsibility upon herself for others' moods and dissatisfaction. Guilt is complicated by the perfectionism that probably results from female gender identity; identifying oneself as inferior (with some kind of hidden flaw) leads to compensating unconsciously. The social devaluation of female caregiving and gender traits continue to contribute to a woman's low self-esteem.

Motivation for personal development is self-initiated through the woman's recognition of her desires "to be somebody." Frequently perfectionism is the presenting problem in therapy at this stage. Aware of both her needs to develop herself and her responsibilities to others, a woman finds that she cannot be consistently perfect in her conflicting roles. The task of therapy is to help the woman discover her personal authority in choosing to be dependent in some situations and independent in others, without internal pressure to conform to perfect ideals across situations.

The therapeutic relationship is more cooperative and mutual now than at earlier stages. Because she is consciously willing to share responsibility for the therapeutic endeavor, the client can form an alliance with the therapist that is ideal for analytical or insight work. This woman can readily develop a more trusting rapport with a female therapist than can women at earlier stages because she can understand gender categories beyond stereotypes. Being able to perceive the social context of female adaptations permits an individual to be more empathic with other women and more confrontive with men. Appropriate tasks for further development, through therapy, include the interpretation of past and present in terms of symbolic themes and the recognition of inner conflict as part of the human condition. Analyses of early developmental patterns, expectations from the family of origin, and "inferior" beliefs about oneself often form the core of therapeutic work. Challenging the client to solve the puzzle of her own identity and offering support to help her develop self-assertiveness and personal preferences are constant themes.

The animus complex usually takes the form of Youth, Hero, or Lover at this stage of development. The ideal of true partnership is emergent in women's relationships with men. Women become increasingly able to rely on themselves for validation of self-worth as they perceive themselves to be equal but different from men. Experiencing animus as Hero involves an active surrendering on the woman's part to her own creative urges and to the development of her own heroic qualities of rationality, endurance, and courage.

There is no chronological period for development of the Conscientious Stage in the healthy female. If it occurs, the stage does not emerge until late adolescence at the earliest. When it emerges in middle or later adulthood, women may be reticent to take on the challenges of their own development. In such a situation they will need additional support from therapists and others in establishing a life context for their personal authority.

Individualistic Stage

The Individualistic Stage is marked by the achieved sense of individuality in a woman's self-concept. The conflicts that the woman implicity felt earlier (at the Conscientious Stage) between her own desire for independence and her responsibility to others will now be consciously articulated. The conflict between personal freedom and interpersonal responsibility is often the presenting problem in female clients. The woman clearly acknowledges the process of psychological development unfolding over her past and is aware of the contributions of early family relationships and female gender identity to her current self-concept. She has developed her own context of meaning for a "life story" that is unique. Accompanying this is her awareness of the frustrations and oppressions she has experienced along the way, as well as a developed concern and empathy for others.

Aware of the essential nature of interdependence in human relating, and of the necessity of attaching to others for her own well-being, a woman suffers conflict over personal desires for achievement and creative expression. She feels caught between herself and the needs of other people. If she has found men to be incapable of cherishing, of caregiving roles, and of feelings of interdependence, she may feel alienated from them.

The therapeutic relationship, which is a partnership of mutual meaning and empathy, can be the ground for strengthening female authority by encouraging and aiding the integration of animus into the woman's sense of self. Learning how to "father" oneself involves the integration of the patriarchal animus complex. The woman learns how to provide material and emotional support for herself in the world and to arrange her family life so that she can achieve a feeling of satisfaction. Often this kind of change will include networking with other women. In addition to interpreting dreams or distortions in the therapeutic relationship, the therapist can offer ideal images of powerful females by suggesting literary, mythological, and artistic sources of inspiration. Female authority figures—goddesses, powerful heroines and contemporary creative women—will enrich the woman's experience of her own developing authority.

The animus complex at this stage of development is the Partner Within: the integration of animus and self in ongoing authoritative and creative activities. Because she has a more reliable source of self-esteem, the woman can differentiate between inner conflict and her own identity. Instead of feeling pulled apart by the demands of different roles she must play, she experiences the freedom of personal authority. She develops an ability to go into the darkness of her own changing moods in order to increase her understanding of her inner conflicts. Because she has developed an attitude of self-reflection and an understanding of the attributions of female gender in our society, she no longer automatically internalizes the inferior aspects of female gender identity. She feels freer to choose her own responses, desires, and attitudes of the movement in most situations.

Autonomous and Integrated Stages

We have combined the last two stages of Loevinger's ego development scheme because the Autonomous Stage and the Integrated Stage depict ego attitudes which are so rare in therapeutic practices as to be only infrequently observed. Women who have individuated to this point are probably as rare as about 2 or 3 in 100. We have met such women in therapy who are struggling to conduct both creative and relational activities in a busy schedule divided between family life and highly individualized work. Their presenting problems usually concern desire for greater insight about some felt conflict, often in regard to intimate relating.

All of the attainments and concerns of the Conscientious and Individualistic Stages continue to be manifest at these last stages. The ability to tolerate ambiguity, to transcend paradox and to engage conflict with humor are the special characteristics of greater reflective understanding at these stages. Such a woman expresses her emotions and insights vividly and colorfully, including her sexual feelings and desires. She expects mutuality and collaboration in the therapeutic relationship and is disappointed when these are not present.

A woman in this stage is actively aware of and struggling with her own conflicts concerning personal authority and empathy. Such a client has much to teach her therapist and may be beyond her therapist developmentally. The woman in this stage cherishes intimate and family relationships more than do women in previous stages. She strives for coherence of personal identity in values and style, across conflicting roles and in her different reference groups. Because she excludes nothing from her potential repertoire of responses in these situations, we can call her "androgynous" in her behavior. She desires a continuous "felt self" that will express her integrity and can struggle with limitations in achieving this desire.

The general work of therapy will consist of helping the woman cope with the anxiety that comes from conflicts between her responsibilities and her commitment to ideals of self-actualization. Much of this work will concern her personal symbolic life rather than interpretations of family-of-origin patterns. The therapist assists the client in examining symbolic motifs and in furthering expression of these through creative work and interpersonal relating. Anxiety about failure is still prominent in such women, and they need to learn to reframe their desire for perfection or self-consistency across competing roles. Supporting the client's humor, reminding her of the broad cultural meanings of her gender and the struggles of women, and reinforcing a variety of different attitudes and approaches will increase the client's satisfaction in living. The therapist's use of self, both in self-disclosure and in interpreting the therapeutic relationship, is essential.

The animus complex that characterizes a woman's functioning at these stages is Androgyne. Although we may not know precisely what this image alludes to, it clearly means a full identity with being human in all its potentials. The integration of masculine and feminine strengths has been depicted poetically, mythologically, and in dream images, as some of our illustrations will show.

If therapy is effective, both therapist and client will eventually recognize an authentic and meaningful interplay of the interpersonal and intrapsychic as different strands of a single process in the development of a unique and imaginative individual.

THERAPEUTIC HELP WITH FEMALE AUTHORITY

Growing older does not guarantee further development or a better relationship to one's animus. Only the continuing struggle to foster a symbolic life and enduring relationships and the riskiness of integrating one's own potentials will lead to progress. The negative self-concepts and low self-esteem that plague women are not simply the products of individual personalities. They are based in the very framework we use to define male and female, and in the symbolic meaning of the division of labor between men and women.

Understanding that the stages of animus development are products of interpersonal and sociocultural relationships with men leads us to focus our therapeutic work on both interpersonal and intrapsychic dimensions of meaning. From the interpersonal side, we attend to the interactive field of therapy itself and to psychological complexes internalized from past relationships and enacted in present ones. Intrapsychically, we are concerned with symbolic transformation of inner images and the progressive development of archetypal emotional expression as observed in dreams and gestural behavior. Neither the interpersonal nor the intrapsychic can be overlooked in any session. Nor can we reduce the importance of the fact that clients go on living in patriarchal contexts that exert pressures to conform to negative female self-concepts.

We encourage all clients to develop a new symbolic context for understanding their personality functioning. Sometimes this entails making "reductive" interpretations that frame the remembered events of a client's past. The patterns or meanings that emerge then situate her primarily in an interpersonal context of her family of origin. At other times, it entails making synthetic interpretations that amplify or expand the symbolic meaning of a particular image, gesture, or habitual action. "Amplification" is a Jungian interpretive method, which refers an image or action to symbolic expressions in myth, legend, folktale, or fairy tale, thereby illuminating meaning without explicit reference to personal history.

Traditionally stories were used to instruct and entertain groups of people. Myths and tales contribute important information about how to function in a human group over the life span. Critical life events—such as infant attachment, separation, initiation to adulthood, territorial dominance, adult bonding, and problems of loss and death—are represented in universal motifs in traditional stories. The characters and situations in such stories tell us how to navigate through expectable crises of human life which affect personality organization and social functioning. Life crises can provide opportunities for further development and increased self-esteem when they are understood as a part of a larger developmental process. They can, on the other hand, provoke stagnation or retreat when they are experienced only as stress or anxiety (see Thrunher, 1983).

Once we have established an appropriate framework for new meaning construction, especially in regard to animus functioning, the client and the therapist can make use of a variety of images and stories from myth and legend to expand the meaning of animus experiences. In the following chapters we have used stories from Greek and Roman mythology to illustrate the emotional significance and dominant themes for each stage of animus development. They provide a context for amplification of the clinical material we present. These stories are by no means the only symbolic contexts we use in psychotherapy, but they are especially good examples of the images many clients find inspiring and useful. In a therapy session, we make use of these images from traditional stories to reveal potential for further development that may be connected to a particular feeling state or unconscious complex. The stories presented here are ones which we have found especially useful for understanding the animus complexes of clients in psychotherapy.

We decided to restrict ourselves to Greek and Roman mythology because they constitute the dominant mythological framework for Western culture. Many of our clients were familiar with these stories when they came to therapy. Furthermore, these stories provide a lens that focuses attention on male dominance and its repercussions. We realize we have risked the possibility that the images of goddesses and women we present are primarily aspects of men's psychology, masculine ideals, or men's relationships with women. We are not offering these stories as ideal representations of female identity. Rather, we turn back to these images to understand how and why women and female ideals have been excluded and repressed. Before we can weave a new fabric of meaning and new forms for female authority, we must extricate ourselves from the old ones and unweave their meanings. By and large, we can assist women in illuminating the roots of their felt inferiority, and in liberating an authentic authority, by turning our cultural images inside out to see what has been hidden or is missing.

We come to these stories with certain questions in mind. What does the story say about a woman's relationship to the masculine in herself and to men in general? What does it say about her relationship with women and the feminine in her own personality? How does the story suggest a direction for further development? In order to study the animus complex in American women, we try to keep in mind the effects of past cultures on our present one. As we review the dreams, fantasies, and strivings of women in each stage of development, we make connecting links between the goddesses of the past and those of the present. For example, Aphrodite is more alive for many Americans in Brooke Shields's ads than she is in Greek stories or even in Botticelli's painting. Images associated with archetypal themes of emotional arousal are linked with our cultural past. Emotional meanings of a client's preoccupations and dream expressions are vivified and expanded through connections between goddesses and gods of the past and popular images and ideas of contemporary culture.

Some explanation of our general method for doing psychotherapy may further clairfy our use of traditional stories. First, we assume (from Jung's theory) that human beings are in a constant process of change or development toward further integration and differentiation. Both in an individual lifetime and in cultural periods, creative experiences bring new opportunities for development. These experiences may be crises. They typically increase tension or conflict between habitual and emergent forms of thought and action. In psychotherapy, we encourage our clients (and ourselves) to become aware of the prospective meaning or creative solutions to life problems that emerge in dreaming and in the interactive process. In order to integrate newly symbolized experience, we may be guided by images or events of a story. In animus interpretations, we can, for example, predict how the complex may be played out in relationship from looking at the different characters and their parts in the story associated with each stage. Again, we emphasize that the stories do not represent ideals, but rather psychological conditions under which we have been operating for many generations in patriarchal cultures.

From the point of view of ego development, we also assume that people carry their own theories about life and meaning. These are somewhat systematic assumptions, hypotheses, anticipations, and ideals. Individuals act in the world based on these notions of self and other. In order to change a person's behaviors, assumptions, or ideals, we must understand and use the client's own implicit theories of life. Archetypal interpretation permits the client and therapist to experience and understand the emotional meaning connected to the symbolic products of the client's ego development stage. A central aim of Jungian psychotherapy is to permit a reconstruction of meanings that are blocking development and new awareness. To assist the client in the unfolding of a new frame of reference—one which permits greater satisfaction and creativity—is a basic objective in our work.

5

Stage One:
Animus as Alien Outsider

The first stage of animus psychology is one of a girl's or woman's containment within her female gender identity. She is enclosed and protected by female power and female authorities. Being Mother and being like Mother are two prominent identity states in this first stage, but so also is being Alien, the Outsider, experienced as the wholly Not-I or Opposite. In understanding the major issues confronting psychotherapy with women in this first stage, we have combined our concern for treating women whose psychological reality remains here due to problematic personality development with our concern for those who remain here due to physical and emotional abuse, in childhood and/or adulthood.

In fact, most clients who remain enclosed in the matriarchal circle of the powerful Mother complex, through adolescence and adulthood, do so because of abuse or abandonment by men on whom they have depended—fathers, older brothers, husbands, uncles, and the like. On the other hand, some women remain within the matriarchal circle because they live within a matrifocal subculture of our dominant patriarchy. Membership is some ethnic groups, especially those associated with southern Mediterranean or Afro-American heritage, includes a prominent identity emphasis in this first stage. Membership in one of these groups can provide a healthy, strong identification with female gender, but it is closely bound to the ethnic subgroup and is not usually an avenue of development in the patriarchal society. Within the boundaries of the matrifocal context, membership in this kind of group is protected by the powers of Mother and female authority, but these are not validated in the dominant society.

Before we introduce the theoretical context for this stage, we want to describe Annette, who presents many of the features of a client at the first stage. At the age of 35, she sought psychotherapy because of a confusing relationship with an articulate woman painter and weaver, a relationship which was apparently dominating Annette's feelings about herself and her own art work, sculpture and painting. Annette found herself accommodating (against her own will) to get the approval of the other woman and seeking out intimate contact in ways which were clearly distressing, constituting what Annette described as a "fixation."

Annette had grown up very identified with her own mother, a woman who had reared five children, visibly giving herself over to each new baby. Annette's father was severe, explosive, and physically abusive to Annette. She had memories of being slapped and beaten that seemed to go back to ages 3 and 4, and potentially included sexual abuse.

Annette had herself been a mother figure to her four younger siblings. In childhood, she had been troubled with a series of obsessions about killing small animals and then about wounding a sibling. In adolescence and adulthood, she discovered she was lesbian and sought intimate, sexual contacts with other women. She evaluated these as frequently uncomfortable and "too intense." She was also troubled by fears of being rejected for being bad, evil, or unlovable, as well as by fears of harming another. In terms of her lesbian adaptation, Annette was ambivalent. She did not feel that she could ever trust a man in intimate relating, but she also wanted to be married and have a family of her own.

At Loevinger's (1976) Self-Aware Stage, Annette is college educated and articulate. She is a promising painter and sculptress who has had several one-woman shows. She is also an able artistic critic. Her employment has not been as interesting or complex as she is. Although she has done some teaching of English in high school, she has by and large held menial jobs (e.g., clerking and waitressing) which are clearly inferior to her skills. She is extremely conscientious about money matters and has been financially independent during her adult years. Frequently she has been anxious and afraid in working with groups of people although she is always a valued employee. In her internalized inferiority, she reflects on herself as an alien outsider and fears that others will reject her as "weird" or too off-beat. Sometimes they do when Annette is too revealing of her inner life or her personal fears.

A sensitive and caring person, Annette is deeply introverted in her feeling responses to others, sometimes appearing aloof and distant although she is wholly connected at an emotional level and hypervigilant about others' comfort. She has a well-developed, ironic humor and can often gain a good perspective on her fears of abandonment and her separation anxiety in being away from those she loves. The following is an example of one of her early dreams in psychotherapy, a dream which illustrates many of the emotional features of this stage of animus development.

I am with some people. I am asking "What can I do? What can I do?" Of course, teach English! I am teaching. I am a man. I am teaching in an alley-way, and I am telling the class that my experiment (no tests, just discussions in which I can tell if they are learning) has failed on several of them. These are the ones of lower intelligence. They even look primitive and dangerous. I look at one who is especially Cro-Magnon-like, and know he is plotting to harm me after class.

I look at myself [the teacher]. I am a man with dark hair and a mustache. A figure appears in a window high above. It is X [a valued woman lover from the past]. She is standing by the window looking out. I look into a window to the right of her. There is a man with blond hair making love to a woman with blond hair. I look back at X again, and see this same man lying on the bed behind her looking at her. She continues to look only out the window. He loves her, but has mischief in his eyes. I look back into the window to the right. The blond woman's lover comes home. He is blond too. He knows she has slept with someone else, and he is in a rage. I know he rips out her gut, but I can only see the bloody knife after the act.

We can associate Annette's experiment in teaching, and her fears, to the beginning of therapy itself in that both she and her therapist were working hard to accept Annette's experience and to "just discuss" rather than test or judge her. Under these conditions of female acceptance, Annette is aware of her "primitive and dangerous" aspects which may harm her after the therapy session is over. In terms of her own authority, she is a man. She has identified with being other, male, when she takes authority, and then she loves the feminine blond woman. The blond woman is clearly in danger from the alien forces of her lover, to whom she has been vulnerable. He can "rip out her gut" and all that Annette will see of this is the "bloody knife after the act." This last scene would be typical of Annette's fear of her own destructive power, the power to kill what is fragile, feminine, and idealized in herself.

Identification with the alien Masculine Other of early childhood can be one of the most troubling aspects of a client's identity at this first stage of animus. When she is in such an identity state or when she projects it onto men, she is wholly beside herself and lacks confidence in her judgments, her own being, and her personal will. Identifying with Mother or Daughter in this first stage is generally more comfortable as long as the presence of anxiety does not overwhelm interpersonal communication. In the presence of anxiety, we will see that the Mother protests, pleads, and demands; and the Daughter is confused, victimized, and lost.

FEMALE GENDER IDENTITY WITHIN
THE MATRIARCHAL CIRCLE

Some theorists, including Neumann (1959), have claimed that even *in utero* identification of daughter with mother, as female and hence same, contributes a developmental advantage to the girl's forming a secure gender identity. Neumann claims that there is a primitive "reciprocal identification" between a female infant and her mother, giving females "from the first the advantage of a natural wholeness and completeness, which is lacking to the man" (p. 67). While this sounds like an appealing argument, we have not discovered sound psychological grounds for assuming that early infant–parent contacts contribute important distinctions to gender differentiation.

Sex-linked biological differences in perception, psychomotor activity, and early cognitive schemes (stemming from hormonal and other brain differences), and early differences in male–female infant handling have not yet distinguished themselves as determinants of gender identity (Money & Ehrhardt, 1972). Gender differentiation involves social cues and language in a way which is dependent on the infant's capacity to construct meanings. Because we are convinced that gender is a product of interaction between biological and social factors, we assume that the earliest period in infancy (from gestation through about 6 months) is marked by a relatedness of self–other which is prior to gender, although parental attributions of gender to the infant are also important in characterizing this relationship.

We take a position consonant with Loewald's (1951) in assuming that the symbiotic or attachment period is prior to the major component of gender differentiation which occurs largely during the separation–individuation process (Mahler, Pine, & Bergman, 1975). During the subphases of this process—body-image differentiation, practicing, rapprochement, and object constancy—the developing infant is gradually acquiring the self–other distinctions which are imbued with gender meanings. Rather than assuming that "normal autism" is the first period, followed by symbiosis, we take the position that the infant–environment dyad is wholly unified in a symbiotic reality which does not include the infant's understanding of gender meaning.

The following quote from Loewald (1951) provides an apt characterization of our theoretical position on the attachment or symbiotic phase prior to gender differentiation.

> The relatedness between ego and reality, or objects, does not develop from an originally unrelated coexistence of two separate entities which come into contact with each other, but on the contrary from a unitary whole which differentiates into distinct parts. Mother and

baby do not get together and develop a relationship, but the baby
is born, becomes detached from the mother, and thus a relatedness
between two parts which originally were one becomes possible. (p. 14)

We assume that the relatedness between "two parts which were originally one" does not become distinctly imbued with gender differences
until the infant is capable of internalized meanings about gender, the
result of language acquisition and certain developmental achievements
of perceptual and meaning construction. This is not to say that the relationship between infant (nonverbal) and (M)other is gender-free, but
rather that the infant cannot participate as a partner in gender meanings until the distinction between self and other (called "object constancy"; Mahler et al., 1975) is clarified. This process normally happens
between 18 months and 3 years of age. During this time, attributions
of "little girl" (little mommy) and "little boy" (little daddy) are beginning to be sorted out as similar to the distinctions between Mother and
Father, between females and males in the immediate environment. We
believe that the earlier distinctions between self and other (concerning
growing awareness of "comfort" and "discomfort" and personal agency) are not gender specific. Although caregivers' responses to female
and male infants are different in quality and quantity from birth onward, these responses do not carry the shared, social meanings of
gender.

   During the phases of separation–individuation, the symbiotic unity
with Mother is likely to be valued differently by girls and boys. Enter
the primary "female relational identity." The symbiotic identification
with Mother is positively valued by the developing girl, and negatively valued by the boy. As Neumann (1959) points out, the female child's
positive identification with Mother can become the primary ground of
personal identity to last a lifetime.

> The woman can remain within the primary relationship, and expand
> and come to herself without having to leave the circle of . . . the
> Great Mother. Insofar as she stays within this enclosure, she is, to
> be sure, childish and immature from the point of view of conscious
> development, but she is not estranged from herself. (p. 67)

   When an adult woman has remained at this stage, she finds the
symbiosis with Mother (usually the parental complex, sometimes the
actual mother) to be the most compelling, powerful, and exciting relationship of her life. If symbiosis with the powerful Mother is positively valued by her extended family and/or her subculture, a girl or woman
may develop without ever becoming estranged from herself. Under
these conditions she will remain enclosed within the matrifocal subgroup and will not achieve power or authority in the patriarchal culture.

Within the family or the household, however, such a woman is confident of her roles and her authority. She is unabashed by masculine
power and unimpressed by men and their work. Within the limits of
her domain, such a woman is grounded in her primary female authority. Outside of the limits, the work belongs to Others. They are undif-
ferrentiated and alien males.

Many women who live within matrifocal subcultures of our society are not troubled by their alienation from the patriarchy. When they
are, however, the focus of their distress is often the men at home
—father, husband, brothers, sons. These relationships may be experienced as inherently different and alien, and they are potentially
abusive. Both the view of male as "alien" and the reality that female
power is not validated by the larger culture can contribute to the victimization of women who remain at this stage. Affective response to
animus, both in self-reflections and in projections, is basic mistrust.
Threats to physical, emotional, and material security of the female are
experienced as basic impingements on identity—whether they occur
via males "on the outside" or animus images within. Feelings of terror, emptiness, dark holes, paralysis, depersonalization, and shame are
the consequences of animus intrusions on female identity. The strength
of trust is within the female bond. Split-off aggression, rage, and hatred
are either unrecognized or associated with love for males, and are
disruptive to continuity of self. Whether a woman is primarily lesbian
or primarily heterosexual at this stage, she may be subject to violent
intrusions of self-hatred which can paralyze her resourceful responses
and undermine her hope.

DEMETER AND PERSEPHONE

The story we have chosen to depict the emotional themes of confrontation with the alien animus is the "Rape of Persephone." It is part of
a cycle of stories comprising the myth of Demeter, one of the earliest
and most powerful earth mothers in Greek tradition. Our concern here
is to illuminate the psychology of animus, both in its early intrusions
on female power (reducing it to "less than male") and in its later intrusions on personal authority. All females living in a patriarchal society
contend with alien animus, just as all female children are "separated"
from Mother by the alien presence of men. Some impingement or intrusion on Mother–Daughter symbiosis is necessary for the process of
individuation; a violent or abusive intrusion is damaging to self-esteem
and psychic integrity.

If actual males in the developing girl's environment are threatening,
aggressive, or abusive to a girl or her mother, then the male Other

(animus) is associated with aggression and violence. The animus complex, as excluded masculinity, remains primitive and split-off as the girl adapts and grows. The complex is alien, unrecognized within the conscious self-image. On one hand, its emotional life threatens disintegration of the conscious self. On the other hand, its occult and mysterious nature may be perceived as exotic and tantalizing. The developing girl is at risk in her attraction to violent, abusive, and criminal men. She is also at risk for feelings of paranoia regarding the partriarchal society, especially its most powerful males, because it is perceived as wholly outside of her strength and understanding. Within the girl or woman herself, her animus perspective engenders self-hatred (when she regards herself from its point of view). Additionally her love for males is mixed with primitive feelings of fear, distrust, and hatred which she cannot differentiate from loving desire.

Her sense of female bonding (the Mother–Daughter symbiosis) is powerfully compelling and (more) trustworthy when she identifies with being Mother or Daughter. Although a particular woman at this stage may not cherish her own mother (she may feel hatred and/or ambivalence because she is unprotected from animus intrusions), she will in some essential way identify herself as Mother or Daughter or an alternating combination of these. In relating to her children, her family members, and her partners, she will feel validated or worthy only in terms of providing nurturant care or in terms of being protected. Ultimately she experiences herself as "belonging to" or being "owned by" these others in a way she finds distressing, confusing, and habitual. Consequently, she may feel it is impossible to separate herself from even the most torturing relationships because they seem to sustain her only access to feeling worthy. She will defend aggressively against separation after she has bonded because these others now seem to be (M)others. The symbiotic Mother may by intrapsychic, interpersonal, or both. Although the woman can consciously observe the destructive aspects of her dependence on abusive and/or powerful others as (M)others with whom she has bonded, she intuitively and anxiously defends against any separation from them.

In the story of Persephone's rape, we can see how the most forceful and intrusive aspects of the animus complex overwhelm a woman's consciousness at a moment when she is reaching out for her own narcissistic needs, her needs to be reflected as a good and worthy person. Just as Persephone is about to pluck the narcissus, interpreted by us as her self-love, she is torn from the bond of her female connectedness.

We quote the following from Carl Kerenyi's The Gods of the Greeks (1974). The story conveys the anxious conflict between naive trust and the force of alien intrusion felt by the girl or woman bound to this stage of development.

Hades ravished the daughter of Demeter, the daughter whom Zeus had given to him without her mother's knowledge. The maiden was playing with the daughters of Okeanos, picking flowers—roses and crocuses, violets, irises and hyacinths—on the lush meadow. Almost she picked the narcissus, too, that flower which the goddess Gaia, to please the god of the Underworld, had caused to spring up, a radiant wonder, as a wile to seduce the maiden with the rosebud countenance. All who beheld the flower, both gods and men, were astonished. A hundred blossoms sprouted from its root, sweet fragrance spread around it, the heavens smiled and the earth and the salty flood of the sea. With both hands the astonished maiden reached out for this jewel. The earth opened, a chasm appeared in the Nysaean Fields, and from it sprang the Lord of the Underworld with his immortal steeds, the Son of Kronos, the god with many names. He set the struggling maiden on his chariot and carried her off despite her wails.

Shrilly she cried out to the Father, the Son of Kronos, the supreme ruler. Neither god nor man heard her voice, not an olive stirred. Only the . . . goddess Hekate heard the cry from her cave; and it was heard, too, by Helios, the splendid son of Hyperion. The Father sat remote from the gods, in his much-frequented temple, receiving the sacrifices. It was his doing that his daughter had been carried off by her uncle, by that commander of many souls, host to many guests. . . . As long as she could still see the earth and the starry sky, the sea and the sun, the goddess hoped to see again her mother and the eternal gods. The mountain peaks and the depths of the sea echoed her immortal voice. The Lady her mother heard it. Sharp pain laid hold of her heart, she tore the head-dress from her immortal hair, cast her dark raiment from off her shoulders, and flew like a bird over land and water in search of her child. (pp. 232–233)

When Demeter finally learns of Persephone's whereabouts and what had transpired, she brings a great famine over the world in grief and mourning for her loss. Her pleas to Zeus for Persephone's release are not attended until Demeter threatens to exterminate the entire race of humans (who bring worthy gifts to Zeus) unless her daughter is returned. At this point Zeus sends Hermes to the Underworld, with a request that Persephone be released. Throughout Persephone's stay in Hades, she has steadfastly refused food and drink, knowing that she will be bound to this realm if she is nourished there. At the last moment before her departure, however, the Lord of the Underworld tricks her into eating a pomegranate seed. Here is how Persephone relates the story to her mother at the time of their reunion.

Whilst they embraced, Demeter was already asking her daughter whether she had taken food in the palace of Hades. For if she had, she must spend one-third of the year below the earth, and only for the other two-thirds could she remain with her mother and the rest of the immortals, returning to them with the spring.

Persephone told how, at the moment when she sprang up in joy to her mother, her husband had secretly slipped the seed of pomegranate into her mouth, and had compelled her to eat it. She also told how she had been carried off while she had been playing and picking flowers. . . . Thus she and her mother passed the whole day, enveloping each other in love. (Kerenyi, 1974, pp. 239–240)

Attachment and separation anxiety are the two emotional states which are depicted in the story of Persephone's rape and her mother's response. These emotional states are central in psychotherapy with adult women who have remained in the early stage of animus development. The Mother–Daughter symbiosis which is reproduced in some manner in the therapeutic relationship, is usually characterized by feelings of anxious attachment. Although these feelings (e.g., heightened concerns about the physical welfare of client and therapist, about the management of impulses, and about basic security) are not present in all therapy sessions, they tend to predominate when the interpersonal field is dominated by the animus complex, the Alien Outsider.

From the story, we acquire certain clues about the needs and behavior of women at this stage. They have, for example, a great hunger for emotional nourishment. (Recall that Persephone takes no food in the Underworld until the very end of her stay.) They want to be seen, encouraged, supported in a nurturant way. There is a concomitant inability to accept and assimilate what is given. (She will not eat the food of the Underworld because she fears it will bind her to Hades.) Anxious need for union with Mother, desire for the security of Mother's protection, and aggressive responses to outsiders are frequently aroused in the intensity of a therapeutic session and are depicted as dream motifs.

STRATEGIES, GOALS, AND TECHNIQUES OF THERAPY

The basic strategy of the therapeutic relationship is to use the empathic rapport between client (Daughter) and therapist (Mother) to support the client's entrance into the outside world of patriarchal culture. After establishing a secure rapport, the therapist will make an alliance with the client against the alien nature of the animus complex.

The general goals of therapy at this stage include the following most prominently:

1. Teaching the client to develop competence in interpersonal relating so that she does not endlessly internalize the personal

stress, agitation, and needs of others as if they were her doing
and had to be soothed by her.

2. Helping the client recognize the meaning of her animus complex
   as alien or threatening to the Mother–Daughter symbiosis; this
   meaning will assist the client in recognizing that she only imagines herself to be flawed, evil, shameful, dirty, or guilty for the
   suffering of Mother.
3. Assisting the client to increase self-esteem by evaluating her
   competence in performing the tasks of ordinary living (i.e., of
   caregiving and concern for environment).
4. Giving the client a variety of learning tasks in which she can
   make contact with the fatherly animus of masculine authority,
   both at home and in the world, in a benign way.

Observation and interpretation of the interpersonal field in the
therapeutic relationship are largely the work of the therapist. Whether
the client has adapted primarily as a Demeter or a Persephone, or has
identified primarily with Hades, she will not show much insight about
her feelings and actions. She is not able to develop a perspective on
her condition. She has no continuous sense of her identity over time.
This is true in the earliest period of separation–individuation (when
this stage naturally occurs) and it is true in adulthood when a woman
has lived primarily within the Mother–Daughter symbiosis. The past,
present, and future do not form a continuous and clear sequence.
Rather, the woman exists in "cyclical time," a nonrational state of being, the repetitive cycles of the natural world, in which the past is
always present and the future is purely unknown.

Consequently an adult woman who has adapted at this stage cannot benefit much from purely insight-oriented therapy. Without other
supports, she cannot examine the past and anticipate the future. She
cannot think about and understand the consequences of her own actions, as separate from the needs and demands of her relational life. She
has not yet assumed a truly personal responsibility in her work or feeling life. She must be held in a corrective emotional relationship through
which she can gradually develop a separate identity as a person.

If the client finds herself in the midst of a crisis of abuse or loss,
she will tend to be blinded by the shock of the moment and need the
assistance of an observing adult (sometimes called the "observing ego"
of the therapist). Because the therapeutic relationship is frequently in-
terrupted by crises, the therapist and client are often frustrated. The
most difficult frustration arises from separation anxiety and concern for
the client's safety. The therapist alternates between feeling too powerful, an idealized being (as the Great Mother) who is expected to protect the client against animus intrusions; and too ineffectual and resisted

(as Hades), one whose interpretations and suggestions are felt as violations or intrusions. Emotionally and metaphorically, the client is hungry for attention. She wants to be "fed," but she displays an inability to take in and assimilate what is given.

The client is suspicious, openly or secretly, of the therapist's reliability and strength. When the client imagines the therapist as Mother, she (client) unconsciously fears that Mother may be impotent if the client falls into hell. When the client identifies with Hades, the therapist is Persephone, who is perceived as confused, helpless, and fragmented. When the client is Persephone, she fears that Mother cannot effect change on Olympus and has no influence (or is in collusion) with Father (Zeus), but makes only idle threats and pleadings. The task for the therapist Mother is similar to the task of Demeter; she must threaten to exterminate all sources of "sacrifice" to Father (e.g., Demeter threatens to exterminate the entire human race) before the client will be convinced of her effectiveness. Again and again, the therapist does battle with the client's impulses of aggression, rage, and envy. Again and again, the therapist contains the client's anxiety about her own right to life.

When there is a traumatic impingement on the client's continuity of being, there is an anxious need to reestablish the maternal symbiosis. Often this means that temporarily the therapist must "think for" the client. Within the traumatic impingement, the client is likely to experience cognitive as well as emotional difficulties. If she has retreated far away from the patriarchal culture, she may not be capable of "formal thought operations" and may need a vocabulary and coping skills for dealing with everyday reality.

Therapy at this stage, then, must occur largely through empathically structured educational activities, advising, counseling, and advocacy for the client's rights. Furthermore, the therapist always presents new opportunities in small portions. (Recall that Persephone eats only a seed from the Underworld of Hades.) Providing the client with appropriate learning tools—through lending books, suggesting activities and workshops, teaching exercises for social skills and self-control—is the practical means for increasing self-esteem and personal authority. These activities are contained within a therapeutic relationship which has a corrective emotional effect on the client. The first phase is a secure *symbiosis* which includes the therapist's attempts to empower the client to separate and "step out" into the patriarchal society. The second phase is the process of *separation* in which the client acknowledges the realistic resources and limitations of her current life circumstances regarding her ability to be an independent person.

During the symbiotic phase, the therapist's major work is containing the anxiety of the client (intrusive animus) so that it does not lead to destructive actions (e.g., addictions, stealing, capitulation to abuse, etc.). Through advice, clarification, interpretation, and support, the therapist provides a boundary for containing anxiety. At the same time, the therapist reflects the authentic worth of the client, a fondness for the client as a person. As the client witnesses her unique goodness in the therapist's realistic appreciation and fondness, the client is able to experience both herself and the therapist as complete and worthy people.

Typically this first phase involves two types of therapeutic expertise: (1) recognition of—and resistance to—idealistic projections of Great Mother or Terrible Mother (projected onto therapist) and (2) acknowledgment of the genuine satisfaction gained from contact with the client. If the therapist senses that sessions are becoming a series of "feedings" of Daughter (by Mother) without notable change in the client, and without felt satisfaction in the work, then the therapist needs to examine her countertransference identification with Great Mother.

As Searles (1965) describes the therapeutic relationship between schizophrenic client and therapist, the "royal road" out of prolonged symbiosis is to go through it. An individual remains within the symbiotic bond with Mother because the person experiences herself as being unable to complete the Mother. When a mother is experienced as tragically wounded or unable to function separately without her children, then the child may remain bonded until the (M)other can be seen as a whole and complete person. It is the worthiness of the child's love which is in question, a love which is experienced as ineffective, flawed, or inconsequential. The schizophrenic person, according to Searles, is trapped within the symbiotic bond because the mother has not been capable of acknowledging the worth of the child, not because the mother has herself provided too little or the wrong kind of love. As Searles (1965) says:

> What happens in such a mother–child relationship as I am describing is that the normal child-love towards the mother is accentuated and, at the same time, blocked in its direction, and turned into complex, indirect channels. That is, the child of a normal mother often feels . . . a desire to express helpfulness and solicitude towards his [sic] mother, especially at times when she is anxious, fatigued, sorrowful, or when she is simply showing a pleasureful readiness for his helpful participation in her work and life. But the pre-schizophrenic child detects in *his* mother—no matter how unable he is to formulate it thus—a tragically unintegrated and incomplete person. To his mother . . . he responds with an intensity of compassion which goes far beyond that which a child would have reason to feel towards a relatively well mother. (p. 231, italics in original)

A Persephone client experiences the Mother complex with this kind of intensity of care, although frequently mixed with fear and aggression. With the Persephone client, the therapist should acknowledge, in realistic and nonviolating ways, the usefulness of the client's efforts to care and be compassionate. During the mutually satisfying activities of therapy, the therapist develops a genuine fondness and respect for the client, feeling the authentic connection of psychological growth together. It is essential that the therapist periodically verbalize the fondness she feels for the client. It is also essential, however, that the therapist resist speaking in false, idealistic, or platitudinous statements. These will only heighten the anxiety of the client who already fears that she will not be accurately seen and/or that she will not measure up to the therapist's expectations. The narrow line walked by an effective therapist at this phase is one of confidence in her ability to validate another person realistically. Naturally the therapist must be able to manage her own narcissistic needs adequately enough to free herself from identifying with idealizing projections and/or fusing them with images of the client.

On the other hand, the therapist also receives hostile and destructive images (primarily of the Alien Outsider) which threaten the rapport. These should be examined without becoming aloof and judgmental (without resorting to the position of Zeus). The client may project the rapist, killer, or abandoning Mother. The degree to which the client is able to express her feelings in words, and then to recognize that they arise in her own internal states, is usually proportionate to the degree to which the therapist recognizes the aggressive feelings as *fear*, the client's fear that her own love is flawed or bad. The client fears that she cannot provide enough sustenance for the therapist and hence will once again be abandoned to her abusive animus. Intrapsychically this fear is a self-loathing, a deep belief that she is neither a good-enough Daughter nor a good-enough Mother.

Through understanding and examining the source of her self-hatred, the client can begin to assimilate interpersonal resources from actual people around her. It is the integration of the negative and split-off animus, in some small amount (only a "seed"), that allows Persephone to remain "above ground" two-thirds of the time. In the story, the seed comes directly from Hades, but can only be assimilated (taken as food) when Persephone is about to be reunited with her mother, when she is about to tell the story of her own abduction.

The assimilation of some aspect of the alien animus comes just at the end of the symbiotic phase when the client trusts the therapist enough to reveal her fears in words. This is the beginning of trustworthy self-reflective thought, the beginning of the symbolic dialectic of formal thought operations.

Again, Searles (1965) is helpful in clarifying the attitude of the therapist faced repeatedly with the client's aggressive hostility.

> In my work with one extraordinarily deeply and chronically ill para-
> noid schizophrenic man . . . I spent the first two years in an osten-
> sibly fully interested and dedicated meeting with him for the sessions,
> consciously making every effort to be useful to him, but, as I realized
> near the end of this period, without his really *meaning enough* to me,
> personally, for me to come fully to grips with the extremely intense
> feelings at the root of his illness.
>
> Not many months later, however, I found that I now cared so
> deeply for him that I was no longer greatly concerned, for example,
> with his long-repeated, furious threats to knock my teeth out; I kept
> moving, psychologically towards him, or one might say remaining
> psychologically available to him, despite these threats. My thought,
> in retrospect, is that he had come to mean more to me than did my
> own teeth. (pp. 240–241, italics in original)

This kind of extraordinary dedication is demanded of the therapist who
creates a container for a Persephone client. It will take time for the
therapist to develop both the trust and the courage to sustain assaults
and acknowledge their actual meaning. When such a bond has been
securely established and can be used as the basis of individuation, the
satisfaction is enormous.

The second phase of therapy is characterized by preparations for
the client to enter the outside world. The client is no longer entrapped
in a frightening symbiotic completion of Mother and she is no longer
vulnerable to profound, disorganizing depression. The continuing use
of educational and self-help resources prepare different clients for different activities. Entering professional or job training, moving from an
institution to a halfway house, leaving an abusive marriage, and becoming less passive in her family are all examples of activities of separation which have characterized our Persephone clients in the final phase.
A woman of 35, for example, moved out of her parental home into a
group home at the conclusion of this phase. With improved social skills
she quite literally left her lifelong symbiosis with her parents. For some
clients, the seed of knowledge (knowledge of her own aggression)
which is swallowed leads not only to increased mastery, but also to increased desire for self-understanding. Some clients remain in therapy
after they have left the Persephone stage; others do not.

In this final phase, the therapist must be aware of her own dependence on the client. If the therapist has identified narcissistically with
idealizing projections, then she will feel especially afraid of letting go
of the client. Even if she has experienced only the authentic fondness
for Persephone, she will be reluctant to let her go. Persephone is genuinely abandoned, however, if she is left dependent on her therapist.
She must herself become capable of life management and some greater
degree of independence. The therapist should support her ability to

actualize her self-interest, make decisions, practice social skills, and get and keep a job—all of these within therapy sessions. In this final phase, then, the point is reached where the therapist puts qualifiers on her love for the Daughter. Urging and supporting practical changes and talking about separation (or changing therapy) is the avenue of individuation. This avenue will increase stress within therapy, and the client is likely to become aware of the therapist as a separate person. The client may dream of the therapist as having too many children, too many clients, having a lover, or doing other things (e.g., eating lunch) during the therapy session. The fear of competition among siblings and the desire to possess the therapist as Mother need to be interpreted and realistically framed as part of the growth process. The client must now be "cut out" of the exclusive symbiotic relationship. Her fears of separation should be acknowledged with a firm empathy. The therapist parts from the Persephone client in believing in her accomplishments and knowing that she can enter the patriarchal world with an ability to compete. Her alien animus complex has been transformed to a fatherly, patriarchal complex, signaling a new stage. The symbiotic fusion of the Demeter–Persephone pair has been transformed into a new adaptation that can be praised and admired in the larger society as a part of the client's independence.

PERSEPHONE AND DEMETER: CLIENT AND THERAPIST

Women who come to therapy as clients in this first stage are usually troubled by the more severe aspects of disturbances of self, disruptions to the sense of being continuous in the moment and over time. In nosological terminology, they are vulnerable to psychoses, personality disorders (especially borderline, avoidant, dependent, and schizoid types), and to affective and eating disturbances (e.g., bulimia) which are related to low self-esteem. Even for women who have adapted well to matrifocal subcultures and generally function competently as mothers, working women, and wives, there may be occasional, disruptive states of "loss of self" and self-loathing due to disorganizing intrusions of negative animus. Difficulty in articulating an identity, feelings of worthlessness, and lack of formal thought are likely to cripple anyone's efforts to establish personal authority in our society.

The Persephone client often is embedded in painful environmental stresses which may seem hopelessly overwhelming. Physical, emotional, and sexual abuse may be in her history—usually the product of her personal relationships with men in her family. A host of needy and dependent people may surround her, and she may not be able to get or keep a job that provides her with financial resources. The imbalance between needs and apparent resources can at first seem very discouraging.

Acting to separate the Persephone client from an abusive environment is the first step in the therapeutic process. Permanent or temporary separation from environmental threats can be a difficult part of the early bonding with this client. Differentiation and separation are the recurring emotional issues of therapy, however, and the initial differentiation of environmental and intrapsychic threats is a step toward individuation.

A client at this stage has many strengths, often not recognized as competences. When she identifies with Demeter, she can be nurturant as well as enraged. She is able to care for herself and others under conditions which threaten survival in fundamental ways. Her identification with Hades can provide adaptive strengths in her incisive criticism, her ability to cut herself out of dangers and to operate courageously within the darker realms of human conduct. One client was able to move quickly in severing the bond of an abusive relationship when she read a book about the cyclical repetitions of domestic violence. This woman had earlier cut herself free of a clinging and destructive relationship with her alcoholic mother. Similarly, the Persephone identification permits the client to speak about darkness within herself and others. Her willingness to see emptiness and the meaning of death (separation from those we love), and to express the pain at being imprisoned in her own fears is an essential strength for developing a full range of meaning in human life. The willingness to encounter pain also contributes to aesthetic sensitivity and interpersonal empathy in Persephone women. They are capable writers, artists, poets, children's educators, nutritionists, and providers of human services which require complex and subtle understanding of suffering. This kind of woman has special skill and competence in nonrational forms of communication and in intuitively judging the meaning of feeling expressions through gestures and nonverbal means.

Although there is no one configuration of parental complexes that holds true across all cases, the one we commonly see in Persephone clients is that of a powerful Mother complex (described as strong, needy, suffocating, or demanding) and an abusive Father complex (described or imagined—in the absence of an actual father—as judgmental, violent, aggressive, or incapable of sensitivity). The desire to love and trust a father has been transformed into hate and rage. Love feelings for men are usually associated with frustration and fear, making the feelings untrustworthy. The consequences of extreme alienation of the animus complex from the conscious identity of the woman–girl are seen in primitive and intense emotional expressions of love–hate, as though the desire to love has been so mixed with fear that it is unreliable as a feeling of love. Holding herself apart and aloof from this alien complex, the woman has tried to adapt to life through a strong self-reliance which may have collapsed frequently into excessive dependence on others.

Leah is an example of a young woman who had "no idea" about her own identity. She entered therapy at the age of 22 and reported depression over her inability to mourn the death of her mother 3 years earlier. At the Conformist Stage of ego development, Leah had made an acceptable marriage and was trying to adapt to society's role of being a loving wife and a stepmother to two children. She had sought approval from authority figures throughout adolescence and was now quite anxious about her husband's criticisms of her. Dan had become bored and frustrated with Leah's incessant needs for attention, praise, and reassurance.

The following dream was reported near the beginning of therapy and depicts a number of emotional themes concerning the unreality of Leah's attempts to be a functional and separate person. Leah and her therapist interpreted the images of the children to be both depictions of her actual relationships with the stepchildren and images of the developing child within Leah.

I picked Dan up at the airport. My father was there and so was my mother. My father's brother was driving the car. We ran into a ditch. I was badly scratched and I cried, "Check and see if Billy [age 14] and Christy [age 8] are all right." We pulled them out and they weren't people. They were long cocoon things. There were three of these things. We opened Billy and he was the darker one. Christy was lighter. They were big worms, like larvae. In Christy's larva, she was cut and bleeding. I was trying to decide if she was alive. I didn't open the third cocoon, but it looked smaller, like a baby larva.

I was looking at the cut: Is she dead? She was alive, but hurt. I didn't know how badly she was hurt or if she was going to live or not.

Leah's association to the wounded Christy larva was that she (Leah) wanted "to get rid of the hurt that's inside." The third cocoon was interpreted as an image of Leah's developing self, whereas the Christy larva had something specifically to do with her own mothering and the Mother–Daughter relationship. Leah experienced herself has having a fatal hidden flaw, a secret fault which debilitated her in a permanent way. She believed that she was weak.

Many Persephone clients firmly and concretely believe they are disabled or evil in some way which makes them absolutely unlovable. They may compensate for this belief by enacting an impersonal servility: Serving others becomes a cover for feeling worthless.

In the story, Persephone is guilty of two evils, offenses against Mother. The first is her narcissistic desire to separate and become her own person. She reaches for the powerful narcissus flower and is confronted by the darkness of animus. The second evil is swallowing the pomegranate seed, indicating by her actions that she desires to return to the underworld, the realm of the male god. The image of an "evil seed" and the memory of having done something terribly wrong are often a part of Persephone's narrative in therapy. Her hidden desire to separate from Mother rule is covered by a conscious belief in her own weakness.

Initially and for some while, the therapist must take seriously and quite literally the idea that the client is fatally wounded. From the point of view of the complex, the client is in grave danger. Protection from the dangerous and abusive animus, protection from self-destruction and others' violence, as well as from addictions and impulsive acting out, are a part of the therapist's initial responsibilities.

Persephone clients do not usually trust the protection of powerful men; working with a male therapist may present an impossible dilemma. Rage at Father is frequently depicted as aggression and violence coming from the patriarchal authorities: Judges, teachers, police, and military officials are frequently portrayed as hostile and dangerous in the dreams of Persephone clients.

Protection by female authority may also be a problem initially. Demeter was ignorant of the plans of Hades and Zeus, and the client fears that her therapist may also be ignorant of the violent intrusions by the animus complex and/or the overwhelming aggressions from men in her (the client's) environment. The therapist, as protective Mother, must look "good enough" to be idealized by the client. For the Persephone client, this usually means "strong enough." It is of paramount importance that the therapist actually appear self-sufficient, healthy, reliable, and whole. The Persephone client will remain hypervigilant for signs of weakness or insufficiency (e.g., fatigue) in her therapist. The client will instantly turn her attention to restoring the therapist to wholeness at such a moment. In extreme situations, the Persephone client has had to focus on saving her own mother and/or herself from the abuse of males, perhaps her own father. She is intensely solicitous in regard to Mother's safety and well-being. She is also vulnerable to a psychotic depression in which she must remain "dead" in the face of Mother's suffering. The good-enough therapist must appear able to activate a change on Olympus and to retrieve Persephone from the Underworld so that her story can be told.

The following dream is from a woman who entered therapy at the age of 23 with a variety of phobias, psychosomatic complaints, and self-lacerating guilt. She was also at the Conformist Stage of ego development and attempting to comply with the concrete, dualistic morality of a Catholic upbringing. She viewed herself as intellectually inferior although she had completed her college education *summa cum laude*. She was employed in her father's company at the time she began therapy. She feared she could not work elsewhere because no one else would want her. Maude entered therapy at the Pandora stage, described in the next chapter, but she quickly regressed to a Persephone orientation when the therapist suggested she leave her father's company. For a variety of reasons, Maude frequently reported that she was "tortured" by her current work environment, where she was constantly under her father's critical eye and felt judged by all of the male employees.

Maude reported this dream during a phase of self-torture in which she was starving herself of nourishing foods and self-mutilating by cutting herself with a knife.

Someone is responsible for murders in a beautiful house where I am living as a starlet. The man is big and frightening and I begin to suspect him. He has a forehead like a gorilla and his eyes are darting around. He is getting very scared himself. I put a coat hanger around his arms and hit him on the head two or three times. I say, "I know it's you," and he says, "You knew it wouldn't be easy," and the man tries to get his arms out and there is a lot of blood around and I am afraid he will kill me too. I push him down a circular hole that goes down a long ways. Then my father comes up. I say, "It was like a situation comedy or *Mission Impossible*" and I am afraid to be alone with my father.

Maude had felt attacked by her father when she entered puberty. He had begun to seem sexually interested in her and at the same time had become quite critical and aggressive in dealing with her. Prior to that time, she had adapted as the Father's Daughter. Just when she needed him for support and reassurance that her developing sexuality and achievements were good, he had turned against her. She felt somehow responsible for this, especially because he insinuated that she provoked his sexual attraction for her. The dream indicates her potential integration of the alien killer animus with a greater understanding of the break in the relationship with her father. The vague killer animus returns as her father.

It is the transformation of the alien animus into the fatherly, patriarchal complex that signals a new stage of development. Better able to survive, the Persephone who can relate her own story is the woman who will eventually become Queen of the Underworld, the conscious woman–self in the darkness of suffering.

6

Stage Two: Animus as Father, God, or King

The major theme of the second stage of animus development is the merging of self-worth with praise, enhancement, and reflections from men. Female gender identity is strongly internalized in its traditional form. The girl or woman believes herself to be inferior to boys and men, and then looks to them for knowledge, guidance, and protection. At this stage the animus complex takes the form of the patriarch: Father, God, or King. If the complex is projected onto the immediate father, it may take on his characteristics. If it is projected onto male leaders or a male god, it can take on both the authority and the aggression of these masculine images as understood from the female perspective.

Because her self-esteem is directly connected to male evaluations, a woman constantly monitors her legitimate value—her truth, beauty, and goodness—in terms of internalized masculine judgments and external male reflections. Thus she regards her best self from an essentially masculine point of view and she always falls short of the standards she applies because she is not a member of the privileged group; she is not a man.

We assume that this second stage begins for most women in early childhood (for some women, later into adolescence or even not at all) when the little girl identifies with the inferior qualities of being female. In rejecting the legitimacy of female authority and in separating from her mother's powerful influence in favor of male authority, the girl has recognized that in our society anatomical differences between the sexes are symbolically equated with strength (male) and weakness (female). What Freudian psychoanalysts have called *penis envy* is an androcentric characterization of this theme. Chodorow (1978) redefines *penis envy* as *phallus envy*—in terms of its symbolic meaning —and says the following about the girl's turning away from female power and toward male validation.

> The penis, or phallus, is a symbol of power or omnipotence, whether you have one as a sexual organ (as a male), or as a sexual object (as her mother "possesses" her father's). A girl wants it for the powers which it symbolizes and the freedom it promises from her previous sense of dependence, and not because it is inherently and obvioulsy better to be masculine. . . . (p. 123)

The attitude about which Chodorow speaks is constructed at the time when the girl or woman is moving into the second stage of animus development. We emphasize that the girl turns away from her earlier identification with female power and authority because she comes to believe that being female means being weak and dependent. It is not dependence that is negative or problematic, but rather the belief that dependence means weakness, and that being female means being dependent.

To have any access to power, the little girl must refashion herself to meet the standards of the masculine order, but she soon understands she cannot become truly male because she does not possess the anatomical qualifications. Her choices for adaptation are to be "like a man" or to be "liked by men," or a combination of the two. She must relinquish her authentic connection to her female experience, that is, to the primacy of female power.

In a variety of ways, she experiences a split between her adopted patriarchal and her original female identities. Turning away from the validity of her own experience is the initial "fall" from identification with Mother. It can be unconsciously imagined as a "sin" or "fatal flaw," which took place at a primordial moment and marked her as inadequate forever. This is especially true if the female later enacts her loss of self-worth in having to submit to humiliating or abusive acts with powerful men (e.g., incest with brother or father) or in deceiving her male superiors by breaking the laws of the patriarch (e.g., shoplifting). If a girl or woman carries out actions, through force or choice, which seem to legitimate her feelings of inadequacy, she is especially vulnerable to long-term, vicious self-hatred. The self-hatred is organized and expressed through a patriarchal animus which convinces her that she is hopelessly evil or bad.

Most women who enter psychotherapy at this or the earlier stage profess some version of the "false self." That is, they declare openly or unintentionally that they have a hidden, shameful core of identity, which has been covered over for a long time by an acceptable facade. They may believe that their cover is a beautiful appearance, graceful decor, charming manner, entertaining wit, or any other version of a feminine mask. Conversely, they may believe themselves to be covered by a pretense of masculinity, a tomboyish attitude, a teasing and challenging manner, mastery of various forms of competition, or some other version of a facade of achievement and success. Finally, if they have adapted both to feminine appearance and masculine challenge, they will see themselves as covering up through constant and incessant performance, assuming a myraid of competing images which are donned in the presence of men. In this third adaptation (the Father's Daughter who is his intimate and equal), the woman sees herself as competing to be most beautiful *and* most successful, on a treadmill of confusing and contradictory activities.

Adapting to male dictates for validation is actually a healthy transition from fusion with Mother to greater independence in a patriarchal society. If a woman remains at the first stage of animus development, she is bounded by the matriarchy whose authority in our society has been limited to domestic affairs and caregiving. In terms of the girl who refashions herself to masculine standards or takes the "hermaphroditic" cover of the Father's Daughter, she is better off than one who is simply beautiful. Identifying oneself in some way with the culturally superior form of authority (i.e., masculine) results in greater self-esteem and mastery, and in less risk of depression, even during childhood and adolescence. A woman who sustains her feminine and weak adaptation well into adulthood will find herself at increasingly greater risk for a profound depression, as her beauty begins to wane with age and the numbers of available men diminish.

PANDORA AND ZEUS

The story of Pandora, in its familiar form from the later Greeks, depicts the fashioning of the first woman by a male god. In Hesiod's version of the story, she is created by Zeus as a punishment for the triumph of men in stealing fire from the gods. If we interpret fire as discriminating consciousness, the ability to differentiate between opposites and to be one's own best judge, then we can say that Pandora's beauty is in direct opposition to it. She is punishment for men's enlightenment and is a representative of all evil. She is nothing but a beautiful appearance who lures men's minds into empty intrigue and into the ways of instinct and nature, as opposed to the ways of masculine culture. This Greek version of the origin of woman is no more disastrous to women's self-esteem than our Judeo-Christian version of Eve, the evil temptress. The Greek version of the story emphasizes the facade of appearance and the Judeo-Christian version emphasizes the quest for knowledge.

The following synopsis of the Pandora story is excerpted from Kerenyi (1974), who summarizes it from Hesiod. The context for the story is Zeus's punishment of Prometheus for having given fire to humans (only men were alive at this point in mythological history).

. . . anger filled Zeus's heart, when he beheld the light, visible from afar, of the fires kindled by men. He straightway prepared for men an evil thing that would weigh equal with the boon of fire. . . . "Son of Iapetos," quoth Zeus, "thou art wiser than all of us, thou rejoicest that thou hast stolen fire and hast deceived me. This shall work harm unto thyself and unto men yet to be. For they shall receive from me, in retaliation for the theft of fire, an evil thing in which they will all rejoice, surrounding with love their own pain." Thus spoke the Father of Gods and Men, and laughed aloud. He bade Hephaestus straightway to mix earth with water, to set in it a voice and strength, and to create a desire-awakening beautiful maiden, whose face should be like those of the immortal goddesses. Athena was ordered to teach her womanly crafts and weaving. Golden Aphrodite was ordered to encompass her head with the radiance of lovely charm and rending desires. Hermes had Zeus's command to fill the figure with bitchy shamelessness and treachery. They all did as the ruler had bidden. The famed master-craftsman fashioned from earth the likeness of a bashful maiden. Pallas Athene adorned it with girdle and raiment. The Charities and Peitho set golden necklets upon it. The Horai wreathed the maiden with spring flowers. In her breast Hermes planted lies, flatteries and treachery. The Messenger of the Gods furthermore gave her a voice, and named the woman Pandora, since all the Olympians had created her as a gift, to the bane of men, eaters of bread. (pp. 216–218)

A well-known sequel to the Pandora story provides another perspective for understanding the complex. In the sequel, Pandora's insistent curiosity leads her to remove the lid of what was apparently an earthenware jar, a receptacle for storing grains or oil. In this jar were kept all sorts of evils—sickness and death among them—from which the race of men had been protected. When Pandora released this "underground darkness" into the world of human beings, she introduced the final distinction between gods and men, that of mortality. Among the evil contents of the jar was one positive element: hope or the belief in a better future. Hope remained in the jar, resulting in some versions of Pandora as a hopeful figure who, like Eve, stands at the juncture between divinity and humanity.

We now remember Pandora largely for having opened this jar, later called a "box." Her curiosity seems wastefully evil to humans who want to be immortal like the gods. Looked at from a theogonic perspective, Pandora's curiosity reconnects her to those powers hidden in the earth, the natural powers of death which relate to her origins as an earth goddess. Pandora's name may well connect her to a more majestic figure as an earlier nature goddess. Her name means "rich in gifts" or "all-giving" and refers to the earth itself (Kerenyi, 1974, pp. 218–219).

Pandora's story provides clues to the psychology of women at this stage of animus development. Her appearance is her only power and it is a negative power. She has been fashioned by the masculine gods as a punishment and a distraction for men. She is apparently caught in the power of her own appearance, which is at the same time evil and her only commodity for exchange among men. Her curiosity about the evils stored underground is commonly understood as a sin. The ability to remove the lid that contains the forces of the buried matriarchal culture (Pandora's lifting of the lid) is psychologically the first desire to penetrate the power of appearance.

At this stage we make no distinction between anxiety over appearance and anxiety over achievement. From the perspective of Pandora psychology, both are facades adapted to the dictates of the patriarchy in order to gain access to patriarchal power. While in a formal or structural sense the animus complex functions similarly with respect to a facade of either beauty or achievement, the adaptive gains of achievement (in terms of actual competence) probably provide greater possibility for satisfaction in middle and later life than the adaptive gains of beauty. The gains of achievement do not so readily dissipate with age, and neither do they depend for their success so completely upon male approval.

TURNING TO FATHER

Turning to Father for guidance into the world, either the actual biological father or the projected animus Father complex, is a betrayal of Mother. The betrayal of Mother is represented in the Persephone story in the plucking of the flower and the swallowing of the seed. In the Pandora story, we simply find that the Mother figure is entirely absent and that the Father (Zeus) demands a female be fashioned according to his dictates. Because Hephaestus is the primary creator of Pandora, we trace the roots of the Mother complex through him, behind the scenes.

Hera gave birth to Hephaestus without the involvement of her spouse Zeus. She created Hephaestus at least partly in revenge for Zeus's giving birth to Athena without her, Hera's, involvement. Hephaestus can be understood as the animus complex of Hera who is the archetypal possessive wife. Hephaestus fashions Pandora, a work of art that demonstrates magnificently his great technical genius.

In mythological genealogy, Hera was first a powerful earth goddess and only later confined to the inferior status of being the wife of Zeus. Hephaestus depicts emotional images that result from confining female power under male dominion. Hephaestus works his ways underground, outside of the Olympian Heavens. Although he is a creative genius, he is not to be included on Olympus, among the gods, because of his low status and his illegitimacy.

The point at which a woman recognizes the limitations of her mother's power and freedom in the patriarchal world is the same point at which she will turn to father or fatherly figures to find access to the power her mother lacks.

For some girls, the transformation of the animus complex from alien to fatherly takes place quite early in development. Gender identity distinctions are usually securely internalized between 18 months and 3 years of age. By the end of that period, some girls have already turned away from the primary identification with Mother and toward validation from Father. For other girls, due to absent or severe or abusive fathering, little trust in males develops in the immediate environment. Although a girl may sense that males enjoy greater freedom and privilege, she continues to identify primarily with the Mother complex in terms of her own identity, while projecting the alien animus complex onto men and boys.

Girls who do not enter into a loving, trusting relationship with a father or father figure will emerge into adulthood without having internalized patriarchal dictates, rules, and values. Unless such young women remain within a matriarchal subculture (e.g., an Italian extended family system), they are at risk for forming an "identity relationship" with attentive and caring males onto whom they project either the Father or the Hephaestian animus complex. In such a relationship, the woman is entirely dependent on the man to sustain her sense of self-worth. She is guided by his ideals, motivated by his standards, and may even achieve through his performances. She seeks protection, vicarious power, and validation through such a relationship. When she is living within the Pandora complex, she finds herself in a round of projections and identifications that take three forms: beautiful but empty evil seductress, frustrated and intense creative genius, and punishing or benign Father. Her chances for breaking out of this cycle and into a greater sense of self-validation and autonomy may be better than for a girl who has become her father's ideal (Father's Daughter) in early childhood, only to be emotionally abandoned in adolescence.

If there is a typical combination of parents that we see in the Father's Daughter form of the Pandora complex, it is the one which mirrors Zeus and Hera. The father is a powerful patriarch or demands to be seen in such a way. The mother is the wife of the patriarch, jealous and possessive of her husband and compensating for his lack of interpersonal skills and competence. The father is usually aloof or demanding and apparently strong. He often has the appearance of the rational male authority: businessman, lawyer, scientist, or physician. He is not approached directly by family members because he is intimidating in a rational, challenging, and aloof way. He presides as the royal father over his wife and children. The mother may be distant and servile, or she may be cheery, gracious, apologetic, and warm. Usually she possesses her husband tightly, whether or not this is apparent on the surface. He is her only claim to status. Underneath her wifely appearance, sometimes quite visible to the world, is depression. She may not speak about it, but her children sense it or assume it in her resistance, confusion, and fatigue. Different from the Persephone complex through which Mother is perceived as strong and firm, the Pandora complex usually includes a weak, ineffectual Mother when the orientation is retained into adulthood.

In the Father's Daughter form of the Pandora complex, the little girl forms an alliance with her father through which she feels her own worth, beauty, or goodness. She and her father seem to share points of views, talents, physical attributes, and values that mother does not share. The little girl feels privileged to be the confidant or companion of her father, although she may feel guilty that her mother has been left out. (Actually an idealized absent or dead father can fill the role of archetypal Father in this complex if the mother is weak, ineffectual, or depressed. The little girl imagines herself to be the close companion of an ideal father who opposes and compensates for the weak mother.) If the daughter's true individuality is not permitted to emerge—either because her father abandons her in preadolescence or because he does not permit differences from himself—then she will retain a highly motivating Father complex. She will attempt to fashion herself according to the dictates of this complex as long as she can project the image onto an actual man or a masculine institution (e.g., Church). The sense of urgency surrounding the need for validation through this form of the animus complex is critical. Without it, as the Father's Daughter, she has no place in the world.

Many fathers actually retreat from their daughters in the girls' adolescence. Because of fathers' fears of sexual feelings for their daughters, the fathers withdraw from intimate emotional contact and/or tease and challenge their daughters in an aggressive way. If the actual father fails to love, protect, and guide his daughter at the critical point of her developing sexuality, the daughter is at risk for being manipulated by powerful, older men.

Freud's (1905/1953) famous case of his analysis of Dora is an example of what we call the Pandora complex. Dora had greatly admired her father, who failed to protect her from the sexual intrusions of one of his (the father's) male friends. Freud's account of this case includes enough information about Dora and her family to allow reinterpretation. Freud reports, for example, that Dora's parents were often in conflict and that each was involved in sexual relationships outside the marriage. Dora seems to have been caught between her love and loyalty to her father and her dependence on her mother. Most Pandora women feel somehow triangulated between Mother and Father, though they are allied with the Father's perspective.

Dora's first dream in Freud's (1905/1953) report of the case seems to depict her father's failure to empathize with the value of the feminine and the contributions of her mother to the family. Here is the dream.

> A house was on fire. My father was standing beside my bed and woke me up. I dressed myself quickly. Mother wanted to stop and save her jewel-case, but Father said: "I refuse to let myself and my two children be burnt for the sake of your jewel-case." We hurried downstairs, and as soon as I was outside I woke up. (p. 64)

Although Freud interprets the dream in terms of Dora's desire to be seduced by her father (and to possess the penis of her father and others), we see the dream as a depiction of the conflicts felt by the adolescent daughter caught in a Father complex. Self-worth, authority, and determination are embodied in the image of the Father in Dora's dream. He directs the movements of the entire family in this crisis and decides what and whom will be saved. The words he speaks to Dora indicate that she perceives him as triangulating her (and her siblings) with her Mother's "jewel-case." Freud interprets the "jewel-case" as the mother's sexual organs. In the absence of Dora's associations, we would assume a more general meaning, that of something valuable and precious to the mother regarding her appearance. Apparently, Dora feels caught between her Mother's jewels and her Father's protection. Furthermore, we can assume that the statement coming from the dream Father means that Dora's Father complex devalues the Mother, whose appearance would seem to be more important than her children's safety. That she would risk her children for the sake of her jewel-case is an indication of a shallow and narcissistic woman. The internal tension between an authoritative and triangulating Father complex and a weak, shallow, empty, or depressed Mother complex is the core conflict of this stage. From other information in Freud's report of the case, we can hypothesize that Dora's father was unable to validate the goodness and worth of his wife's contributions to the family and to society. He denied his wife's contributions to the family and to society. He denied his emotional dependence on his wife, and he had betrayed her. Internally, Dora is compelled to seek approval and acceptance from an authoritative man partly because she cannot ally herself with a weak, narcissistic Mother. In order to survive, to be protected from critical intrusions on her sense of integrity, Dora allies herself with her Father complex and opposes her Mother complex, leaving her with the experience of a "false self" covering a weak, empty, and fearful true self.

Adult women who have remained in the Father subphase of the Pandora stage must continually restore their self-esteem through male approval and reflections of their beauty, worth, or intelligence. If the woman's adaptation has been to identify with a beautiful appearance, she may seem to be a parody of femininity. Exaggerated concern for makeup, hairdo, jewelry, or physique is typical of this kind of adaptation. Identifying with the power of appearance is more adaptive to a patriarchal culture than is fusing with Mother in the Persephone stage. Beyond young adulthood, however, life becomes a series of desperate efforts to defeat the process of aging. What began as wanting to be feminine turns into a mad rush from beauty salon to exercise spa, or from love affair to love affair, in an unconscious effort to maintain self-worth. Caught in a vicious cycle of appearances, the aging Pandora woman must now resist looking inward, opening the dreaded container of her internal female suffering. Her appearance has come to stand for her only power. It has provided material rewards and emotional gratifications which seem irreplaceable. She fears that she cannot learn to develop her own competence and authority, a relationship to her own creativity and inner life. She fears the reality of grief and mourning over lost possibilities. And indeed she is loathe to abandon the only perceived control she has securely achieved, control over her appearance.

Here is a dream from Lucy, a woman in her early 30s who had become extremely skeptical of any woman who was not feminine in her manner.

I am a butterfly. I touch down and up. I fly free in the sunshine. I fly to the sky and then I soar and sit back down on a flower. I am warmed by the sun. I feel mostly peace and freedom where no one can pin you down and no one trap you.

When Lucy entered therapy, at the Conformist Stage of ego development, she identified her problem as her husband. He was a "dull drag" on her exciting and dramatic life. That she perceived him as unsuccessful in his business and mediocre in his ability to compete was her stated reason for feeling low self-esteem. Lucy knew that she often felt incapable, wounded, and depressed, but she could not identify these experiences with anything about herself. They had been completely projected onto her husband. She was herself a beautifully groomed, appearance-oriented business woman. She competently managed a clothes business and kept her house well decorated, an apt showcase for her own beauty. Like some other women at this subphase, Lucy consciously assumed that life should be "one big party" and that work was a burdensome means to a desired material goal. What began as a desire to please her Daddy and to share in his material success and social influence had become a cover of dramatic beauty, a stimulating self-enclosed hauteur. Lucy was extremely skeptical of looking beneath her surface to uncover any ugly or wounded parts of herself. She hoped that her adaptive cover would hold her together until she could remake the "disappointing" man onto whom she had projected her Father complex.

Her power was not self-engendered and therefore could not be securely reliable. Because she pressured her husband to carry her own needs for financial and social status, she attempted to control his performance in the business world. His failures in this area of his life were most distressing to Lucy, far more so than anything in her own personality.

Another client, Maddy, exemplified a frequent feature of the Father subphase of Pandora: the suspicion that "all of this is mother's fault." Her emotional desperation of compensating through appearance is conveyed in the next dream. Maddy was 28 years old when she entered therapy and she had achieved a Self-Aware ego orientation. She reported serious concern about her dependence on her boyfriend and about her extremely negative feelings for her deceased mother. The mother, a wan model-like figure, had died of cancer when Maddy was in her mid-20s. When Maddy entered treatment, she was pursued by a recurring fantasy that her mother was rotting in Maddy's bed upstairs in her present home.

Blaming mother can be interpreted as a daughter's conscious or unconscious recognition that she (daughter) has been carrying aspects of her mother's Hephaestian animus complex, her mother's unrealized creativity and achievement. Whether the daughter identifies with this complex through appearance or achievement, she will have a sense of carrying out the mother's wishes regarding aspects of her own (the daughter's) personal life. Consciously the Pandora woman usually describes her mother as having been too weak or incapacitated for accomplishment in the patriarchal world. In other words, the woman who remains at this stage well into adulthood tends to see her own mother as deeply flawed, and usually complains about her mother not having stood up to her father.

The Pandora woman in the Father subphase demonstrates many wifely and feminine strengths, but she does not affirm them in herself. They are empty, inferior, or stupid activities. This woman is pursued by inner terrors about her hidden flaw. Eating problems such as bulimia, fasting and overeating, are connected with the problem of a fatal or hidden flaw—an emptiness within. In order to soothe the anxiety of low self-esteem, this woman "feeds herself" or "starves herself." She may feed herself at one moment as self-soothing and then loathe herself for having eaten. If she vomits to undo her offense against appearance, she will tend to describe the vomiting as a relief and a self-control in "getting the poisons out." The anxious treadmill of ritualistic activities built around eating, elimination, exercise, and right appearance can be exhausting and hopelessly depressing. These activities function as unconscious confirmation of the belief that a woman's self is indeed secretly damaged, stupid, evil, or weak.

In the case of Maddy, she had given up trying to "look like mother" years before and had instead turned to overeating for solace. Maddy assumed that her mother was sorely disappointed in her daughter's appearance, a disappointment which was compensated for (from Maddy's point of view) by her mother's avid hopes that Maddy would become a concert pianist. Her mother had indeed wanted to be a musician herself, an aspiration she had abandoned when she married.

Over several years, while Maddy's mother was ill with cancer, Maddy had troubling fantasies of her mother's skin cracking and flaking, worms emerging from the cracks. Soon after the mother's death, Maddy had the following dream:

I walk into the den and father is dead with two marks on his neck and blood dripping down. Mother smiles eerily and has fangs. She says he's sleeping. She starts walking close to me and says that she wants me to come close to her and hold her to prove my love to her. My brother runs in the room and says "Here, here, take this stake. Mother's a vampire." I want to kill her and I can't. When I wake up she is near my neck. She is repulsive. She wants physical contact. If I give her that I am more vulnerable. If I prove my love to her, I'll lose myself.

Maddy's mother had provided adequate care and love for her daughter. But her mother's only power had been appearance. The daughter doubted all of her mother's encouragement for Maddy to accomplish something with her life because the mother seemed so disabled herself. "How can Mother know anything about the world out there when she has never done anything with her own life?" is the query of the Pandora daughter, so that rather than embrace her mother's advice, such a daughter is suspicious of whatever the mother offers, even love. Instead the daughter heeds the Father or her patriarchal animus complex. The complex is represented by the brother in Maddy's dream. The brother and Maddy conspire to save Father from the dreaded vampire Mother. Maddy's dream images are a painfully clear depiction of the split between the daughter and her Mother complex. If the daughter embraces this negative, wounded Mother, she will lose herself. Often the daughter has confused the negative Mother complex with her actual mother. Furthermore in opposing the Mother complex, the daughter necessarily identifies with the patriarchal powers. In Maddy's case, as is common, the saving power of the patriarch was first projected onto her own father, who was willing to carry it, and then onto her boyfriend, who was not willing.

Here is another of Maddy's dreams which illustrates how painfully she has split off the evil feminine from the good and strong masculine in herself and her relationships.

A group of people are pursuing me, male and female. The only face I could see was my brother's. I run into a room and against the wall. They were evil people pursuing me, demonic, like hell. They felt and looked evil. I slipped and fell down and my brother grabbed my arm. I said, "Lord please take me now." My body became an iridescent glow, like pure white. I was looking down at myself and felt happy I had died and wouldn't be evil.

Experiences of depersonalization, dissociation, and disidentification with the body can occur in extreme situations of negative self-regard.

Dream confrontations by crowds of examiners is another common theme. They may be confronting the dreamer for real or imagined failures, about secrets or demands. Maddy's dream may indicate a secret incest wish or an actual incest occurence. Incest with a brother can be a dimension of this stage, whereas abuse by the father or an older man is more commonly an actual occurrence for women who remain at the Persephone stage. For Pandora women, sexual accommodation is the focus of response to male demands. The female experiences herself as passively accommodating rather than actively responding. If a girl or young woman does actually give in to incestual or otherwise abusive sexual demands, she will have unfortunately provided "justification" for self-condemnation.

GOALS, STRATEGIES, AND TECHNIQUES OF THERAPY FOR THE FATHER SUBPHASE

The ultimate aim of therapy at this stage is to free the client to look inward and to pursue the objects of her own curiosity. To do this she must reunite in some manner with her female authority. A woman therapist seems to be important in this process. A male therapist with a feminist orientation can also be helpful, as long as he is clearly free of projecting his own negative Mother complex and/or anima demands onto his client.

The first requirement of therapy with such a client is for the therapist to present herself in a very professional way. The client will scrutinize carefully the therapist's appearance: her attractiveness, grooming, office decor, etc. More than at other stages, the way the client perceives her therapist is important to the therapeutic relationship in order for a "good-enough" mothering to take place. Since the major motif is the opening of Pandora's box, the client is intuitively assessing the power of the therapist to make this step safely. The client assesses appearances, in terms of beauty or achievement, the only valid assessment she has known.

The second major concern in therapy with a Pandora woman is her vulnerability to being rescued. She will insist on remaining passive, on being imprisoned by the father and on being unable to identify with the mother. The therapist should be wary of responding to questions like "What should I do?" when they are asked early in the therapeutic process, before the client has taken any responsibility for her therapy. Only after a full map has been made of the Father and Hephaestian forms of the animus complex can the therapist respond to these questions without being hooked by the client's animus.

The movement in therapy is toward the woman's reunion with female power, authority, and curiosity. Experiencing directly aspects of her own competence and freeing her actual mother from the weak, negative complex are prerequisites to opening Pandora's box. The therapist must be especially careful to resist every temptation to side with animus assumptions of female or feminine inferiority, especially those masquerading as supports for adapting to the patriarchy (e.g., Isn't it really better to go to medical school and become a psychiatrist than to go to social work school and become a social worker?).

Subphases of therapy with a woman at this stage typically evolve as follows.

Forming an Adequate Rapport

Here the therapist must ally herself with the client's frame of reference in an objectively empathic way. That is, the therapist must be able to intuit the validity of the client's reasoning about patriarchal standards without validating these standards. A neutral attitude about the actual values, coupled with a deep compassion for the woman's suffering, is generally an effective vehicle for rapport. The therapist should especially attend to looking lively and seeming to be strong, reliable, and convincing.

Confrontation with the False Self and the Parental Complexes

The Pandora cover or false self has been built according to the demands of the parental complexes, in compensation for Mother's weakness and in identification with Father's (or another man's) strengths. Usually the masking personality is defended by rather immature adaptive mechanisms. *Projection*, attributing her unacknowledged anger and aggression to others, whom she then distrusts (especially women), is usually prominent. *Hypochondriasis*, the unconscious transformation of aggressive impulses and fears of abandonment into complaints of physical illness and fatigue, may initially interfere with therapy as the woman genuinely believes she is incapacitated in the face of life's demands. (Naturally a therapist should suggest that physical complaints be examined by a physician for potential somatic problems.) *Passive-aggressive behavior*, in the form of acts of self-harm, procrastination, and/or failure, is often present in some major aspects of the client's social or occupational functioning. Finally, *acting out* of anxiety through impulsive gratifications (especially through alcohol or sex) must be monitored throughout this second phase. Acknowledging and taking responsibility for the anxiety of low self-esteem is the core issue.

Engaging the Authentic Female Self

The client experiences direct contact with her own feelings and the strength of her female self. In this phase, the client should be encouraged to experiment along new lines of her own creativity regarding her life issues at hand. Learning how not to retreat defensively in the context of patriarchal demands, or in conflict with masculine authority, is one element of new learning that should be engaged. The client's intelligent decision making and curiosity are awakened both within and outside of therapy.

When the Pandora client can see that the adaptation to appearance, made by herself or her mother, is an exploitation of dependence eventuating in shame and guilt, she can be freed from the belief that her shame about hidden flaws refers to something literally true. Even so, the client has suffered real losses of opportunities and relationships because she has identified herself as inferior. Unless the client can develop a symbolic connection to her own development and comes to a new creativity or a new understanding of shared community with other women, the client may continue to experience herself as lost. This third phase of therapy, engaging the authentic female self, should be under the direction of the client's own initiative and shaped by her own curiosity.

TAKING ON GODS AND KINGS

Paradoxically, this subphase of the Pandora complex depicts a personality that is both more open to connection with symbolic meaning and more severely self-destructive than the fatherly forms of the animus complex. The adult woman who has this kind of personality typically has remained at the Persephone stage of development into early adulthood due to absent, distant, or severe fathering. She has not developed an adequate loving relationship with any trustworthy male in childhood or adolescence, but she has conserved the Father archetype in its ideal form. Due to her mother's strength and protection, or to the benign nature of her father's involvement, she has not abandoned trust in men. Through her own power of appearance or achievement, she has differentiated herself from the Mother–Daughter symbiosis. With a liberating belief in her independence, beauty, or intelligence, she turns enthusiastically to the patriarchal authorities to fill the place left by the father. She projects a suprahuman power onto the masculine forces in her life, which capture the vitality of her animus complex in the image of the creative underground genius (Hephaestus) or the powerful male god (Zeus).

A woman in this subphase has turned her attention away from the personal world of mothers and fathers and toward the abstract masculine concerns of aesthetics, rationality, religion, politics, or similar preoccupations of patriarchal society.

Three symbolic themes are common in the dreams, fantasies, and activities of women in this subphase: cleansing or purifying the self of a basic flaw, self-sacrifice to spiritual forces or spiritual experiences, and confusion between sexual and spiritual connections to males or authority figures. Adolescent and adult women search for ideals and beliefs that will release them from inner experiences of inferiority and self-hatred, that will transform a negative self-image into a more positive ideal of sacrifice.

From our clinical experience, we have come to believe that young women who have not been validated by fathers or similar paternal figures are most at risk for fragmentation of self at the Pandora stage. The early lives of such women did not permit the humanizing of the archetypal Father image, which has been conserved in its ideal form as part of the animus. In such a condition, the animus complex is infused with suprahuman images and sublime ideals. Due to the woman's low self-esteem and her intense projection of vitality, worth, and creativity onto the male, she may come to relate to her lover in ways that are actually inferior, humiliating, and belittling of herself.

A typical case of this sort is the college woman who is feminine and intellectual, who has been sustained throughout childhood through a maternal circle of support and empowered primarily through her relatedness to women. She has not been abused or overtly punished by the males around her, but she has not been cherished by them either. Her entrance into the patriarchy in college is marked by her own aesthetic and intellectual achievements. She is "ready" to take on the world of men.

Her animus complex is the epitome of spiritual asceticism in its demands for her to be perfectly beautiful, honorable, truthful, etc. Her first direct authentic intimacy with a male friend or lover takes the form of a disintegrating, passive sacrifice of herself. She sees the man as far more beautiful, intelligent, and exciting than she can ever be, and she pursues him obsessively. Her pursuit of the masculine Other has the form of an addiction, as Woodman (1982) puts it, an "addiction to perfection." Under these conditions, she may confuse sexual experience with spiritual conversion and imagine her lover to be a god.

The next dream is that of a 20-year-old woman, a Catholic working-class girl, who had been fused with the Mother complex (in both positive and negative forms) and reared in a matriarchal subculture until her entrance into college at the age of 18. At the age of 19, Patty experienced a profoundly disintegrating identity relationship with a young man, a musician onto whom she had projected the genius of a great composer and the beauty of a god. When Patty lost the relationship (which had been ambivalent at best from his side) at the age of 20, she had retreated into a morbid state of self-abnegation and humiliation. Through meditative practices, dietary restrictions, and overexercise, she hoped to become the perfect partner to this lost lover, who would then rescue her from despair. At the Self-Aware Stage of ego development, Patty was cognitively complex and had previously been self-initiating in her goals for her own academic and career development (goals which she had cast aside in the throes of the relationship). Her dream, about 4 months after the bitter end of the relationship, was vividly recalled:

I am standing in the doorway, looking through a glass into the backyard of the house where I live. My best girlfriend is standing in front of me. Outside everything is a mauve fog, very eerie. The fog is moving about and some of it coalesces into a giant ghostly form. It is huge, manly and frightening. From the distance, the form moves toward us. Just before it closes in, a male voice says "Destiny is a man." My friend drops dead. I wake before it gets to me because I know I will die also.

The animus complex, in the form of what Neumann (1959) calls the *paternal uroborus* or the undifferentiated power of abstract masculine spirit, has been directing her destiny. Patty experiences its force as deadly in the dream and understands its message as death to the female self. The dream is a startling depiction of the emotional intensity of this masculine, spiritual threat to the developing identity of the young woman. Looked at from a progressive developmental perspective, the animus is demanding the death of her attitude about men, the death of her passive femininity. Gradually, Patty was able to reshape her sense of self around realistic goals and to enter into less demanding relationships with men.

Another case was less successful in outcome. A 23-year-old woman, a Lutheran from a middle-class family, entered therapy with complaints about being nonorgasmic. This girl had grown up in a traditional Lutheran family, where her considerable academic and athletic achievements had received little attention from her admired father. He was aloof, commanding, and dramatic, and focused his hopes for future family status on the accomplishments of her two older brothers. In adolescence, the girl felt herself to be bright but unattractive, of little use to her father, and was fearful that she would not marry and bear children, his only wish for her. One afternoon at a church youth group meeting, when she was 13, she was instructed by an attractive older boy on performing fellatio. After that first experience, she began to compulsively perform fellatio secretly on different men and boys. She kept this compulsive activity as a dreadful secret, revealing it to no one, over a 10-year period. She found it very difficult to confess to the therapist, but now made her own connection between the activity and her inability to enjoy intercourse. She described the activity of fellatio as disgusting and humiliating, but she was anxiously drawn to perform it two or three times a week. Although she no longer believed that this was all she had to offer men, she still was excited by the reports of her partners that she was a great lover and a beautiful, sexy woman. In her mind, this humiliating activity had become associated with bowing before a man—before God himself—and making herself humble. She found some spiritual gratification in the image of humiliating herself for men's purposes, but also wondered if God had denied her the pleasure of genital sex as a punishment for some basic and unknown flaw in the core of herself. Because she had concretized her own feelings of inferiority, and found some secondary gratification in the anxious expression of her impulses, this woman found genital intimacy with men very difficult. The death of her mother, just prior to therapy beginning, and her continued financial dependence on her father, mediated against the restoration of her female authority. This young woman left therapy with a sense of self-condemnation, a depressing belief that God had not yet released her from her punishment for having a dark seed within. Both her Conformist ego functioning and the gradual sacrifice of her own college studies seemed to keep her locked into an absolutistic splitting of good and bad elements of the world, and her own identification with the inferior aspects of the split.

In terms of deficit diagnoses, women in this subphase may be classified as having dysthymic or cyclothymic disorders, narcissistic and histrionic personality disorders, eating disorders, and anxiety disorders such as phobias and panic attacks. Absolutistic thinking—a splitting of good from bad values and influences—may protect a woman from encountering her own depression and anger. She identifies with the bad and evil, while projecting the good, worthy side onto the masculine Other. When the Other takes the form of a distinctly male god, the dictates of religious practices may create a barrier to further development.

The critical and judgmental animus is harshest at this subphase. The voice of the complex is a belittling, distant, demanding, judgmental male voice. It judges coldly and demands perfection. The woman has the experience of something in her that watches vigilantly for errors, flaws, ugliness, mistakes, and stupidity. Her own orientation to herself is that of deficit thinking. She assesses herself only in terms of what has *yet to be done*. What she *has accomplished* and how she *now appears* are empty of any real value for herself.

The effect of this kind of complex on her relationships with other people, even other women, is deeply troubling. Self-doubt and emotional detachment are evident in her manner. She can isolate herself from all intimate relationships because she believes that her influence is so inherently negative. Under these conditions, her perfectionism may overtake her ability to treat others compassionately. Intolerance of her own weaknesses leads to intolerance of others' mistakes. She may withdraw into a bitter and cold self-denial in which her anxieties gradually become somaticized as cardiac complaints, vomiting, fatigue, and body aches.

The strengths of this type of woman are numerous. She is assiduous in her pursuit of perfection and therefore has acquired skills and knowledge in a variety of areas. Hardworking, she usually adheres to established conventions about the best ways of doing things. She is especially good at handling structure and organization of tasks and in rallying herself through anticipation. Her "future" orientation has both useful and harmful side effects. On the useful side, she can serve herself and others by planning in advance, monitoring diverse variables, and devoting herself to details. She is well suited to activities that involve planning and providing services: teaching, nursing, human services, legal professions, business, and politics.

GOALS, STRATEGIES, AND TECHNIQUES OF THERAPY FOR THE GOD SUBPHASE

The major goal of therapy with a woman at this subphase of the Pandora complex is identical with that of the Father subphase: The woman must be freed to look inward and pursue her own curiosity. Physical

appearances and rescuing are not major problems within the therapeutic relationship as they are at the other subphase. Rather, the therapist will be challenged along the lines of intellectual, spiritual, or
political performance. The therapist must appear to be on the right side
of the issue raised. A Pandora client has underlying trust neither in the
process of therapy nor in her own ability to become empowered in a
patriarchal society. In her own way, she will insist on the theme of her
imprisonment and look to the power of the therapist as the method of
escape.

The three periods of therapy involve challenges and strategies to
combat the godly or kingly animus that are slightly different from those
involved with the fatherly animus complex.

Forming an Adequate Rapport

Confronting the client's hypercritical and judgmental attitudes toward
herself in a compassionate way is part of the first phase of therapy. The
therapist allies herself with the female identity of strengths and competences, and helps the client reflect on the unreality of her perfection-
istic expectations. Reflecting on, listening to, and exploring responses
are usually the best avenues for making an empathic bond with the
client's female identity. For example, a statement such as ''It sounds
like you believe you should protect everyone in your family from any
discomfort'' is more effective than ''You appear to be overcontrolling
in the face of anxiety.'' Allying oneself with strengths and revealing
these in the context of true limitations of personal responsibility will
open the door to an examination of the general perfectionism of this
client.

Confrontation with the False Self

Internal feelings of emptiness and lack of structure will predominate
in the confrontation with this client's Pandora image. Rather than reflecting the parental complexes *per se*, the godly adaptation is more
stringently held to abstract masculine standards of beauty, truth, ideals,
etc. As described earlier, the defenses against the underlying feelings
of emptiness and loss are usually immature: projection, hypochondriasis, passive–aggressive behavior, and acting out. Passive–aggressive
defenses predominate in this client. She may need close monitoring
of self-harming, self-abnegating behaviors during this period as she
confronts the false self. The client may experience the therapist as trying to take away the only structure on which the client can rely: her
standards for right and wrong (however distorted these might be).

Dream material can be espeically useful in showing such a client how promising her situation is and how her inner life is not as empty as she would imagine.

Here is an example of a dream of an overweight woman in her early 30s who entered therapy because she feared abandonment by her male lover. Although she was at the Conscientious Stage of ego development and could reason about her own feelings and ideals, Wanda felt quite lost when exploring her failure to relate to men intimately. Her adult life had been riddled by interpersonal losses that had been truly beyond her control. Irrational guilt and self-blame about these losses, as well as her haunting perfectionism, supported her facade of being nurturant and cheerful. The following fragment is a part of a dream in which Wanda is taken to a foreign country, and is on a precarious cliff where there is no support underneath. The cliff is hanging over the ocean. The scene includes a group of people, and a machine that is making predictions. Here is the last scene of the dream:

When I attempted to reach out and grab the balcony, the cliff started to give way. I caught the balcony and all the other people fell into the ocean, and the cliff with them. I told everyone to remain calm. I was being interviewed and they wanted to know what happened to the others. Because I wasn't ready for it, the technical team had arranged it so I would understand how it felt to fall. Even though I wasn't ready, it felt all right somehow.

The technical team and interview could be understood here as a part of Wanda's therapy in which she was asked to look beneath her facade of nurturing as well as into her despair over "never attaining anything" for herself. Well-timed and effective self-disclosure on the part of the therapist can be helpful in assisting this kind of client through her fears of emptiness and lack of support within. The more destructive fears of dark holes and emptiness that accompany borderline psychopathology may emerge during this period of therapy. Sometimes the critical identity issues of the Pandora stage and legitimate fears of parting with a Pandora adaptation (e.g., regarding losses of socially condoned power, such as competition for beauty among women) prolong the disintegrating anxieties of this subphase of the complex.

Feelings of being cut off from oneself and one's sexuality may be manifest. Actually these feelings are common complaints of women who enter therapy with a godlike or kingly animus. Sexual contact has often been reduced to a "husk of meaning," as one client called it, an empty shell without any satisfaction.

The following dream offers an image of this experience. The client, April, was in her mid-30s when she entered therapy. At the Conscientious Stage of ego development, April had mothered three children and supported her husband's career in the first 15 years of their marriage.

Now she had returned to graduate school herself, seeking her PhD in a therapeutic profession, but she was "trying not to rock the boat" of her marriage. In other words, she was continuing to be responsible for all of the chores and activities of her marriage, while taking on graduate courses as an additional burden. April was apologetic about her self-interest in pursuing graduate studies. She acknowledged her exhaustion and emotional depletion, but she would not claim any limits to her own self-reliance. April described her inner state as cut off from vitality: "I feel when I lie down and cry that unless there is someone to hold me, I will fall apart." Here is a dream she had at the point of confronting her false self:

I was in a surgical room, like a gynecological examination room. My husband was there and I noticed that his hair was perfect. He was the doctor, and he was sewing up my vagina and saying "It's because you don't need it." He could do these things, but it wouldn't stain him.

The focus of this phase of therapy is a realistic confrontation of the limits of human responsibility, performance, and energy. Regarding the Pandora facade, the ideals of perfectionism have been incorporated through some form of punishing demand, whether positive (for greater perfection of appearance, spirituality, or performance) or negative (for greater humiliation and mortification). Until limitation is understood and loss is adequately acknowledged and grieved, the therapist must maintain a watch on the real strengths and competences of the client. By claiming and internalizing the skills and knowledge she has actually achieved, the client can strengthen her female sense of self and validate its worthiness. In essence, the client is achieving a perspective of her own on the world (integration of animus) which is realistic and female.

Women's support networks, educational tools (such as cassettes and books), and creative activities that strengthen female validity are very useful in working with Pandora women who are not incapacitated by loss in confronting the false self. When depression is prominent, a corrective emotional relationship with an accepting parent–therapist, who soothes and guides the client through her depression, will take precedence over supportive and educative means of increasing female authority.

Engaging the Authentic Female Self

The client is encouraged to explore new lines of development in the issues of her life. The key concern for the therapist is to help the client distinguish between attitudes of self-sacrifice and true personal satisfaction in pursuing her own development. When a woman feels such satisfaction, she can perceive and validate the strengths of her beauty, accomplishments, and skills in a way which is free of harsh animus criticisms. This does not mean that the woman is no longer self-critical, but rather that her self-criticism is not defeating or abusive. In her daily life, she no longer feels compelled to appear or achieve in a narrowly defined way. Also, she feels free to engage in collaborative relationships with other women, and to validate her own mother—without compulsively seeking male evaluations of these activities. Similarly, she no longer automatically suspects herself or other women of being manipulative, inherently weak, deceitful, or overcontrolling.

To say this another way, we see that the woman no longer competes with other women solely for men's attention or patriarchal rewards. She does not view herself primarily in an opportunistic or self-protective competition with women for scarce available goods.

Here is another dream from Patty (whose dream of "Destiny is a man" was reported earlier). Patty reentered therapy (after having been in therapy for almost a year after the breakup of her identity relationship with the musician) in her early 30s. She was still working through the Pandora stage of development, now wrestling with the problems of engaging her authentic female self. At this point, Patty was married to a man considerably her senior and was the mother of two young children. She had recently returned to graduate school to pursue a doctoral degree in psychology. Like April, Patty was pursuing her studies in addition to maintaining her household and mothering her children, while trying "not to rock the boat" of her relationship with her husband. At the time of this dream, Patty was functioning at the Conscientious Stage of ego development with some movement toward Autonomy. In adolescence and early adulthood, Patty had been a perfectionist in her academic achievements. At the time of the dream, she was preparing to take qualifying examinations and she was consciously motivated to complete this task in a new, more adult manner. She did not want to be driven by her belittling godly animus. The main character in the dream is Dr. R, a well-known psychologist who was one of her professors. Dr. M, the man in the film, was an internationally recognized scientist whom the dreamer did not know personally, but whose work she admired.

I am in Dr. R's class and he asks me to describe or define some concept and is very critical of my answer. Slowly he tears it apart, pointing to one flaw after another and asking another woman in the class to provide an alternative answer. The other woman, a better student, does so enthusiastically.

Dr. R is quite fat and the classroom is also squat, a little like the inside of a spaceship or a flying saucer. I am seated in the front of the class.

I am humiliated by this display and feel that R has purposely snagged me into a trap in which he has determined, from the start, to show the faultiness of my thinking. Now I have revealed myself as a fool, falling into the trap. I also feel that I am being played off against this other woman student, who is my rival. I try at some point to reply to a question that seems misleading and designed to trap me further. My answer is dismissed by R with a wave of his hand.

Then he tells us that he has brought a film to class: "Dr. M in Space." The projector is turned on and there is Dr. M floating in space in a starry night sky. He is wearing a silver space suit, which has an orange urine tube coming out the front like a neon umbilical cord. He is simply floating around, while the narrator describes his current research on outer space. I am very distracted by my feelings of humiliation. I turn to a young man seated next to me and say, "Well I *must* know something. I got an A+ on my paper in here." The man says, "Yes, I guess an A indicates something," but does not seem convinced. I look up and see that Dr. R has left the room and will not be available to talk after class. I wake with a very uncomfortable feeling.

The dream shows the conflicts the dreamer feels about competition with women, validation by male professors, and the spaced-out or ungrounded quality of her critical animus. She attempts to validate herself but uses only male standards (i.e., the A+ on R's paper and the reflection of the young man next to her). The dream helped this woman see the essential importance of assuming a more collaborative, noncompetitive attitude with other women students. She experienced abandonment by the godly animus (Dr. M), who was like an infant floating in space, and by the kingly figure (Dr. R) who simply set the trap for argument between women but was not present to work through the differences. Actualizing herself on the grounds of her own existence—graduate school and family life, in this case—meant forming more collaborative relationships with women like herself and finding ways to be authentically present, even during examinations.

The ability to act in one's own favor and in one's own defense, even if acting anxiously or ambivalently, gradually proves to the woman that she will not fall apart without male approval or support. The main task for the therapist working with a client in the final phase of this stage is to help the woman become more self-supportive and affirmative as she pursues the objects of her own curiosity. Strengthening positive self-evaluations and self-interest along realistic lines of development results in a new feeling of freedom for the client. She begins to understand that her needs are worthy of attention and that she is valued for something other than "being a man" or "being liked by men."

The goal for which therapist and client are striving is the opening of Pandora's box, the look inward at the suffering, shame, loss, and anger connected with having lived primarily through masculine approval, through a false self. To open the lid to one's internal life as a woman in a patriarchal society is the beginning of a new stage of development.

7

Stage Three: Romancing the Hero

The Big Bear Man: This man, unknown to me, is a male type that I am always looking for—relaxed, accepting, loving, quiet, nonverbal. Big thing is his solid rock quality. He is *there*, to be depended upon, sprawled upon. You can go to sleep in his lap, and even active little boys . . . are soothed by his charm. With this Big Bear Man, I could survive, live.

—Dream passage from a Psyche woman

The later stages of animus development begin with the image of man as Hero. The heroic man is admired for his strength, his courage, and his ability. He is the prototype of the man whom the woman at this stage "would like to marry." He is fashioned from her own heroic animus complex and does not exist in the world of waking life, although the woman is initially quite unaware of this. Indeed he represents such high standards (e.g., "rationality and justice" or "compassion and sensitivity") that he may best be thought of as an ideal, that is, as the epitome of patriarchal virtue.

The heroic animus may not represent itself as a man at all in the minds of some women; rather it may be manifested as a desire to accomplish goals in the world of men, such as earning a higher educational degree, fighting for social justice in the legal system, or restoring successful functioning to a weak and failing business. The real test of courage will come to the woman at this stage when she must satisfy her masculine ideals by joining in some kind of contract with the patriarchy in order to achieve her individual contribution to society. She may falter or fail at this point if she feels that she has "nothing to offer" in exchange for partnership. A woman who does enter into an heroic partnership, however, and who perceives herself as good enough to be in a bargaining position, tends to be self-affirming and usually anticipates certain outcomes—for example, to be cherished and protected by a man in exchange for what she will contribute. Only with the understanding that her needs will be met, will she embrace the Hero.

This embrace signals a new kind of developmental event: A man and a woman begin to share equal worth out of need for each other. In a patriarchal society, the image is typically interpreted as the romantic embrace of marriage, a social institution dominated by males who subordinate females and dependent others. Naturally, a woman is at risk both socially and psychologically when she embraces the heroic animus in a society that draws limits to her equality with men in both private and public life. Consequently, we find that women experience this initial embrace as a "death marriage" or a "leap into darkness." Whether a woman embraces her ideal lover or her ideal career, as she takes this step toward conscious recognition of her own mastery, a challenge to her ability to be an agent in her own life will emerge.

Eventually, a woman at this stage will focus on the meaning of her work. Her useful activity and her creative self-expression are the nourishment for her psychological growth, although the woman may be completely unaware of this at the time of the initial embrace. In a recent informative study of mastery and pleasure in middle-life women in America, Baruch *et al.* (1983) discovered the following as their "most important finding":

> In the past, a woman's love life, her age, and whether she was or was not a mother were considered more central to her life than her work. Our study shows that these aren't very useful in predicting a woman's sense of pride and power—her Mastery, in our terms. But the relationship between paid work and Mastery . . . shows . . . how vital a role work plays. (p. 103)

They discovered that paid work, especially work which challenges skill and imagination, contributes most importantly to a woman's sense of mastery in middle life.

Entering the workforce may not be primarily on the mind of the woman who contracts for partnership with the patriarchal Hero, but the ideals of work (involving determination, courage, intelligence, authority, and competence) eventually become the subject of her struggle. Marking the end of the stage is the woman's "inward journey" or deepened self-reflection, which includes consciousness of the limitations of both her appearance (as social power) and her ability to be effective as an agent in a patriarchal society. She must understand her own development and her contribution to the culture. Constraints on her roles and androcentric assumptions of her inferiority must be examined in the context of her own personality—that is, what she has internalized from her socialization. Her completion of the stage is signaled by confrontation with the meaning of these and acceptance of her own heroism, especially in response to the suffering of women. The integration of the meaning of female identity results in a shifting of her attention to the restoration of female authority in herself and in the society.

HEROIC COMPLEX AND THE DEATH MARRIAGE

The major emotional theme of the third stage of animus development is active surrender. In contrast to passive sacrifice of self-worth and self-interest at the Pandora stage, this woman willingly gives herself over to the patriarchal forces in an effort to make a contract of equality and shared responsibility for her own pleasure and survival. She will provide or perform in certain ways for men as long as they promise to cherish her and provide for her. The contract is actively pursued in the belief that heroic males (whether they be lovers or professors, ministers or lawyers) have in mind the best interests of women and others over whom they hold the power of truth, beauty, and goodness.

What is the form of the heroic animus in the imagination of the woman? Typically this complex has the agentive and intellectual, and the ethical and aesthetic qualities which have been excluded from her best self. The complex is imaged in terms of her most cherished ideals, which are yet unrealized in her life. If these are artistic and creative, then her animus promises genius in this area. If they are rational and ethical, her animus is projected in that direction. If she does not complete the development of this stage, but remains within the partial achievements of the death marriage (i.e., the unconscious embrace of animus), then she will attain only partial images of her masculine ideals.

A woman who remains at this stage throughout her adult life will have a variety of identity projects underway which embody her ideals, but she will not have secured a primary motivation to bring them to completion or closure. For example, she may do some creative work in her spare time without taking her creative expression seriously enough to discipline herself. Moreover, she will experience herself to be what Claremont de Castillejo (1973, Chap. 4) calls "Woman as Mediator." Although Claremont de Castillejo assumes that a woman's inherent role is to be mediator to a man (or men), we believe that a strong woman remaining in this stage vicariously rejuvenates her creativity through this role of mediation. Her self-worth is predicated on her ability to inspire the creative, thoughtful, ethical men around her. It is the psychological development of the other (her child or partner) that is the vital life project of such a woman. She will, however, continue to be frustrated because she cannot engender in others the qualities she so admires. Similarly, she will tend to mourn the loss of her own greater potential for mastery as she assists others in developing theirs.

The heroic complex is endowed with a mixture of abilities and skills that permit people to enact their own lives as doers and makers. These are aspects of competence, which by definition is the opposite of helplessness or depression. Seligman (1975), in his famous study of "learned helplessness," has shown us how profound and fundamental a human need competence is. Without what Seligman calls "perceived control" of our lives, we tend to resign ourselves to apathy, stagnation, or even death. Aspects of mastery and competence which have been unintentionally excluded from a woman's identity, but which are admired by her all the same, comprise her heroic animus complex. For most women in adulthood, this complex is also fused with aggression and anger. In proportion to the extent a woman has repressed and projected her heroic animus, she will have feelings of resentment and rage at having been "denied" the right to experience her own competence.

A major developmental task at this stage, then, is to differentiate aggression from responsibility. Initially a woman fears the aggression she feels in her own masculine identity; she may imagine a vindictive "macho" destructiveness in herself—the product of splitting off her own legitimate authority from her sense of self over the years. Increasingly, as she experiences the difference between power and authority, between control and authenticity, she will recognize her female authority as humane, personal (i.e., not omnipotent), and valid.

We believe that female aggression tends to be, in any case, different from male aggression in terms of the images presented in dreams and fantasies. Female aggression is depicted as poisoning, casting magic spells, wielding small knives, stone walling, name calling, and stagnation (as anger turned against the force of life). We find these images connected with the female self far more often than scenes of rape or bold killings in the dreams of women we treat at this stage.

We interpret the themes of darkness and fearful anticipation to be connected with repressed and undifferentiated aggression, resentment, and rage in the woman. In order to discover her own heroism, she will have to encounter her own aggression and it is this challenge that she most fears.

AMOR AND PSYCHE

The story of Amor and Psyche, taken from a version (Grant, 1962) of Apuleius's account in *The Golden Ass*, provides us with a rich array of identity images for the heroic stage of animus development. These im-

ages, as at the other stages, may be projected, repressed, or unconsciously identified with. The major characters in the story are Amor,
Psyche, and Venus. The story is told as follows:

> A king and a queen have three beautiful daughters. Much the most
> beautiful is Psyche, the youngest. People come from many lands to
> admire Psyche with the belief that she may be Venus herself, or may
> have replaced Venus as the Goddess of Love. Venus is very angered
> by this and poisons the hearts of Psyche's suitors so that Psyche is
> thoroughly rejected by men. In the face of his daughter's beauty,
> Psyche's father suspects that something "divine" has gone awry in
> that no man wants to marry his daughter. He goes to consult an
> oracle. Venus responds to him at the oracle that his daughter is
> destined to marry a monster, a winged serpent of whom even Jupiter
> is afraid. He is told that Psyche must dress in the black clothes of
> mourning, on her wedding day, and go to a distant mountain-top
> for her death marriage.
>
> To the accompaniment of funeral music, Psyche leads her wed-
> ding procession like a woman going to her grave. Left by her parents
> at the top of the mountain, in dreadful fear, Psyche is lifted by a gentle
> wind and carried to a grassy, flowery field. When she lands there,
> she looks around and sees a palace of gold and gems, and unbe-
> lievably valuable treasures. She enters the palace, believing that she
> is perhaps dead and that this is the palace of a god. Here she is un-
> dressed and bathed by invisible hands. Then she is fed marvelous
> foods and pampered in every possible way by the invisible hands.
>
> Night comes and she falls asleep, but is awakened at midnight
> by a gentle whispering. She is afraid, knowing that anything might
> happen in a vast, uninhabited place like this. She fears for her chasti-
> ty. In a whisper, the gentle voice of a man tells her that this is her
> husband. The unseen man embraces her tenderly and makes love
> to her. She is very satisfied. The man tells her that he can come only
> at night and that she will not be allowed to see him, but that all of
> her needs and desires will be answered in the palace, by day and
> night, as long as she does not try to find out who he is.
>
> At first Psyche accepts her lot willingly, amazed by the splen-
> dor and riches of her palace. Soon, however, she longs for her parents
> and her sisters, and begs her husband that she be allowed to return
> to them for a visit, in order to reassure them of her safety and good
> fortune. Reluctantly her husband agrees to her request, instructing
> her to remember that she can neither know nor reveal his identity
> or all will come to an end.
>
> Psyche returns to her family and relates the story of her marriage.
> Her sisters, jealous of her good fortune, persuade her of the necessity
> of discovering the true identity of her husband. After all, they tell
> her, he may be a monster and she may be endangering herself by
> surrendering to him.

On her return to the palace, Psyche is determined to have a look at her husband and afraid that her sisters' suspicions about his dragon nature may be true. Armed with a candle and a knife, Psyche welcomes her husband on the night of her return. After he has fallen asleep, she grasps the knife and lights a candle. The god Amor is revealed in all his beauteous glory. Psyche is so astonished by the beauty of her husband that she carelessly drops some hot wax on him. He awakens, curses her, and flees. From atop a cypress tree, Amor reproaches her for her thoughtlessness and then soars up into the air. He must return now to his mother Venus, never to mingle with another mortal woman.

Psyche is remorseful and begins to wander about the earth in search of her husband. She comes to a temple of Venus. Now enraged by Psyche's beauty and by her alliance with Amor, Venus sets some impossible tasks for the young daughter-in-law. Each task involves a feat that is apparently impossible for a young woman to perform.

Although Psyche is much discouraged, she ventures out with faith in her great love for Amor. At each step of her heroic adventure, Psyche is assisted by some aspect of nature or the world around her.

Her final task, the most difficult by far, is to fetch a box of "beauty" from Proserpine (Persephone) in the Underworld. Declaring that Psyche is herself a witch, Venus bids her to take an empty box to Proserpine with the request that the Queen of the Underworld fill it with her own beauty in order to restore the appearance of the aging Venus. Venus states that she has faded in beauty due to the exhaustion of nursing her ailing son. This time Psyche is helped by a talking tower that instructs her on the exact steps for getting into and out of the dangerous Underworld. Returning with the box, about to have satisfied the quest for her lover, Psyche is tempted out of foolish desire to have some of the beauty for herself. She is confronted by death, which Proserpine has secretly placed in the box, and falls into a fatal sleep.

Seeing his lover thus, Amor pleads with his mother that Psyche be made immortal and come to live with him in the heavens. Eventually Venus agrees and Amor fetches his bride, rescuing her from a death sleep, and returns with her to the heavens. (summarized, not quoted from Grant, pp. 357–362)

We present this story in such detail because it provides a context of psychological nuance that is remarkably subtle and accurate for understanding women at this stage. First, the surrender of Psyche—leading her funeral wedding march—is a compelling depiction of the ambivalence and fear with which the woman anticipates the consequences of her partnership with the heroic man or institution. A willing surrender of a woman's hopes and needs in exchange for a contract with the masculine forces beyond herself is indeed dangerous, yet she actively goes out to meet her destiny, despite her fear or dread.

The Psyche stage begins with a reactivated fear of the powers beyond oneself, especially a fear of the masculine monster one has unknowingly created within. Some women about to marry find themselves inexplicably asking themselves, ''What have I gotten myself into?'' The fear of marriage is a fear of both the patriarchal powers encroaching on one's freedom and the aggression of one's own identity needs (mastery and competence).

The realistic fear of socially sanctioned male aggression must also be emphasized in our study of the ''death marriage'' theme. From the research of Maccoby and Jacklin (1974), Whiting and Whiting (1975), and Bardwick, Douvan, Horner, and Gutmann (1970), we learn that both within our society and across cultures boys have higher activity levels, are physically more impulsive, are prone to act out aggression, and are more aggressively competitive than girls. If girls consistently accommodate this level of aggressiveness in boys and men, the associated experiences, images, feelings, and concepts contribute to the aggressive nature of the animus. Most patriarchal societies encourage males to translate physical activity into aggressive and competitive forms of interaction. Confusion between aggression and authority, as embodied in dominant males, is a by-product of such societies. Because certain males dominate by imposing their will on others, and heroic males (i.e., leader, teachers, and managers) may seem empowered by aggressiveness, a woman necessarily fears to surrender herself to partnership with them. All her experience tells her it would be too easy to become overwhelmed or overpowered by masculine authority.

The relationship between woman and animus differs significantly in each of the three stories we have presented to characterize the self-animus dimension of female identity. In the Persephone story, a young woman was victimized by a sudden rape or intrusion through which she is unwillingly bound to the dark realm of a destructive animus. In the Pandora story, a woman is literally created by powerful masculine gods who are vindicating their own authority over humans. In the Psyche story, a young woman actively enters into her own adventure, which has been arranged to punish her for competing with the goddess of beauty, the ''old mother,'' Venus. Psyche's fearful and aggressive (i.e., bringing a knife) investigation of the masculine god results in a direct confrontation with the negative Mother complex. Competition between mother and daughter, jealousy among sisters, and confrontation with the underground power of the female (Persephone's box of beauty, which actually holds death) are the central motifs of aggression in this story. The challenge of female aggression and the fear of male aggression are foci of the struggle for greater individuation. (Obviously the Psyche story is related to Cinderella, a variant on the same theme. The fairytale of Cinderella somewhat belies the seriousness of the depression and rage that arise in the process of restoring female self-esteem.)

The potential for regression to earlier stages of animus development is depicted in Psyche's underground descent and in her wish to indulge in the "eternal beauty" of Persephone's box. Identification with beauty as power necessarily leads to death (i.e., depression, helplessness, stagnation), because it brings a woman into direct confrontation with the raging goddess, her Mother complex. She will feel constricted by limitations of her gender identity, misled by androcentric definitions of her personal worth, and painfully aware of the confinement of her mothers in earlier generations.

The desire to look into the darkness of her arrangement with men (i.e., Psyche's lifting the candle to see Amor) is a dangerous desire, sometimes provoked by jealous sisters who are themselves at the mercy of unconscious urges. The inward look into the character of female identity must be supported with a fundamental understanding and confidence in one's own worth. If there is no such foundation, a woman may remain captured by the resentment, bitterness, and loss that she encounters in her darkness.

Psyche's desire to have some beauty for herself can also be interpreted as a final challenge to the Mother complex. Psyche's self-interest results in a shocking loss of her old idea of herself and in her subsequent transformation into a goddess. The story does not end until the old Mother has accepted her new Daughter as an equal. Although Amor pleads for Psyche's rescue, it is not the power of Amor which is active here, but rather a benevolent recognition by Mother that Daughter is strong enough to possess her own female authority. The psychological connection between the heroic animus (Amor) of the woman and the negative Mother complex (enraged Venus) has been an unconscious collusion. As a final development, the woman must free herself from the domination of her Mother complex, especially the envious and embittered attitudes toward other women it embodies, yet remain able to understand and join with her heroic animus.

In order for this to happen in the most optimal way, we have come to believe that the woman must claim her femininity as worthwhile, whatever her adaptation has been to the category "female." This means that the woman comes to recognize her contribution to culture and society as intrinsically valuable in whatever feminine form it has taken: greater empathic skill in relationships, a strong and reliable aesthetic orientation, an altruistic desire to provide care, etc. Through this kind of self-regard, the woman is finally able to form an equal partnership with men and with her animus. The resolution of the heroic stage is the recognition that men are "male persons" without a *magic* power or authority intrinsic to their gender. No longer does such a woman seek primarily to emulate men, to be approved by male institutions, or to belittle other women for their adaptations.

STRATEGIES, GOALS, AND TECHNIQUES OF THERAPY

The basic therapeutic strategy at this stage is to increase the client's responsibility for her own life. This strategy must be fundamentally grounded in empathic rapport so that the therapist can clearly see and accurately interpret the client's competences, both potential and actual, while challenging passive dependence on male approval or judgments. Interpretation of parental complexes and of the animus complex (especially as it is currently projected onto men in the client's life) is the central technique most useful to increasing personal responsibility in a woman at this stage, while identifying and carrying out tasks of new learning (another basic strategy of therapy) is secondary.

The goals of therapy at this stage can be summarized as follows.

1. The basic aim is to assist the client in differentiating her own needs, desires, attitudes, and aspirations from those of the significant men in her contemporary life, and from those unexamined attitudes of her Father and Mother complexes.

2. Consequently, the client should show an increase in actively claiming responsibility, achieving competence, and/or expressing creativity in the work of her daily life. Within the area of her material support (income and the like), the client must confront and understand the meaning of her own life choices whether these have been toward material dependence or independence, toward nurturance or achievement. A part of this process will involve the client and therapist understanding the limitations and losses involved in the client's contracts with the patriarchy. (There are limitations and losses in all such contracts.)

3. Conscious integration of the meaning of losses regarding material dependence should lead into an analysis of disappointment, anger, and/or aggression in the client's relationships with men, other women, mother, and father.

4. Realistic identification of creative areas in the client's current work life should enhance both pleasure and agency. Ideally, the client should have some opportunity to increase her sense of self-worth and to accrue greater reward (material and/or emotional) from her efforts. This constitutes the final process of differentiation of the heroic animus and the withdrawal of its projection onto men and/or male institutions. As part and parcel of this process, the client will experience

an increase in courage and skill in using the resources of her culture and society to meet her needs.

5. The final goal of therapy at this stage is differentiation of the Mother complex—both positive and negative—from the actual mother: The therapist and client move toward affirming the client's actual mother as an individual who struggled for her survival within a particular life context. This process includes a confrontation with the meaning of female gender identity, in terms of the mother's circumstances and identity choices.

6. Increasingly the client can use the analytical and intuitive skills gained in therapy to understand her own images, metaphors, dreams, longings, wishes, and disappointments. In achieving such an ability she develops a working knowledge of the ongoing dialectical relationships within her personality and life situation, between herself and her animus complex.

Although a woman entering therapy at the heroic stage of animus already perceives herself as having something to offer, she may not be sure what that something is, and she may interpret it differently on different occasions. Sometimes, for example, she thinks it is nurturance and at others, insight. Whatever the bargaining chip, she has surrendered or wants to surrender it to a partnership of equality, but she sees the masculine other as more powerful, intelligent, aggressive, etc., than she is.

The following is a dream from Linda, a 46-year-old woman who is an accomplished professional. Linda had been actively involved in advocating for women's issues although she had secretly resented "tough feminists" and found herself often in alliance with men on certain issues having to do with family decision making. Her presenting problem in therapy concerned her inability to form trusting relationships with men. She had been married briefly when she was in her 20s, but the marriage had ended disastrously when her husband collapsed into a profound psychotic break. Linda often feared aggression in the men around her and quite unintentionally developed an "entertaining manner" in response to her fear. Her dream:

At church, at a meeting, a woman brought two dishes of lovely donuts, some coated with colored sugar and some with brown sugar. Then two women walked in, women whom I know. One was D and the other was an attractive, dramatic woman who seemed familiar. They wanted to ride home and I said "yes." Suddenly I was next door to the church in a dark area, waiting for a train. I saw some young Black boys, around six or seven of them, go by and I was a little frightened, but watched them. D had said "Don't go into the dark alone" and I suddenly remembered her saying this. I waited until the train left and crossed the track. I was going up to a building when a young man grabbed me. I was so frightened. I tried to yell and no voice came out. Then I said to him "What are you doing? Stop this." And I am not sure what he said. We struggled and suddenly we were inside the building in the light. These students were around and no one was taking me seriously. I finally began to calm the young man.

A younger woman friend approached and I asked her to watch the young man while I called the police. He said something to the effect that he didn't really know what it was to "fuck" (I am not sure he used that word) because he "couldn't get it up." I said that was usually connected to the rage he felt at women, usually the first woman in his life. He said, "Yes, my mother." I looked at him. He was white, in his early 20s and clean cut. I held him a minute and felt sexually attracted to him. I told him he needed therapy and I wanted him to come to church with me. He could be helped. I said, "In fact, either you do that or I call the police." The feelings seemed caring on my part, bewildered on his.

Earlier in the dream, I had been on some department store tour on which I had gone at least three times. I wondered why I didn't do something else. A lawyer friend was there and I called her over to ask how her mother was. She said "O.K." and that she had just seen her. Her mother was in a rest home; somehow her father was going to give her mother money, but then realized it was too expensive. Perhaps the woman was another friend, but whoever she was she had just been to the U.S. Supreme Court to argue. She had gone in and told the men she was there. Just as she was ready to go in, they broke up the session for refreshments. She was disappointed and wanted to go in. People, largely men, just stood around and talked, and she was frustrated.

At the Conscientious Stage of ego development, Linda had been in psychoanalysis and psychoanalytic therapy with male therapists for 18 years (almost continuously) prior to entering therapy with one of the authors. During this time, her male therapists had never seriously questioned her dependence on them for a close male relationship, even though she was sometimes in frequent psychoanalysis (i.e., three or four times per week) and in no other regular intimate contact with male companions. She indeed had strong romantic wishes regarding most of her male therapists and had been quite openly seduced by one of them.

Her entrance into therapy with a woman, about a year and a half before this dream (therapy occurring once a week), precipitated some deep distrust of women professionals. Although she was quite eager to begin with her new therapist, she found it difficult to trust the expertise of a woman. This attitude allowed both therapist and client to examine some of her assumptions about women, especially about women professionals like herself. At the time of the dream, Linda was working on a new creative project and had freed herself from some of the rigid constraints of her earlier unconscious male orientation.

Typical of the beginning of the Psyche stage of development is the occurrence, in fantasy or dreams, of gangs of male hoodlums or rowdy boys—or sometimes groups of critical male professors. The aggression of these animus figures is not as frightening or overwhelming as alien rapist or killer figures of the Persephone stage.

The dream begins with the "sweet" nurturance of women and the dreamer's connection with her feminist friends at church. Linda had enriched her life through new connections with women friends and had acquired an attitude of trust; she believed the warning "Don't go into the dark alone" (reminiscent of Psyche's sisters instructing her to take up a candle in the darkness of her romantic love). The animus figures who appear are less threatening and more playful than at earlier stages. The aggressive qualities the woman fears are not as difficult to confront as she imagines. Her own masculine aggression is represented first in "splinters" or collective fragments of male groups which eventually become transformed into a more unified heroic vision for her life. In the dream, Linda looks closely at her attacker (i.e., brings him into the light). She discovers a rather attractive male, who speaks to her about rage at Mother and its consequences for his love life.

Many Psyche clients enter therapy both with a sense of confidence in some of their abilities and with a challenge to the therapist's expertise—especially if the therapist is female. Linda was clear about her professional accomplishments and she was apprehensive about trusting a woman therapist, although she was herself a professed feminist. We believe that the major difficulty for the female therapist working with the Psyche client is the challenge to the therapist's identity. The transference relationship most frequently lived out is envy between Mother and Daughter, and competitive rivalry among Sisters. If the therapist has not penetrated her own relationship to gender identity issues, such as appearance and achievement, then much confusion can arise. The confusion between the "invisible hands" of the nurturant Mother (regressive identification with passive dependence on Mother) and the challenge of the new therapist Mother (as a role model in the client's ongoing life) is problematic at this stage. If the therapist holds an ideal, consciously or unconsciously, that passive dependence is a promising goal for an adult woman, then some kind of depression will consume the therapeutic relationship. If the therapist acts as Great Mother or too aggressively opposes Great Mother orientation, she will contribute to the client's hopelessness about struggling against passivity (either in relationships or work). Although a woman may be cared for in the most splendid ways (by her nurturant women friends and/or by her husband or father), she will neither experience the confidence of self-control nor understand the connections between her own actions and their consequences (contingent behavior) until she has herself mastered the environment on which she depends. Personal autonomy or power is not the goal of this process, however. The goal is personal authority in knowing how to make one's own decisions for greater life satisfaction.

Usually the Psyche woman is enraged (identification with Venus) or depressed (identification with Psyche at beginning of story) when she enters therapy. She has recognized and validated her own self-worth in some ways (not challenging the patriarchy, but assuming its validity). Yet she cannot see how her own competence has ''done her any good.'' She may have been betrayed by her husband, overlooked by her boss, or rejected by her children. She feels that the conscious awareness of her situation she has already gained (that she is facing a dangerous precipice and an impossible conflict) has been won at a great cost. She may indicate that she can no longer trust men or women, or believe that women can exist in their own right—or, especially, trust the enthusiasm of younger women that ''women's liberation'' will bring any greater ease for anyone. The ideals of liberation seem like a sham and the burdens of responsibility seem somehow overwhelmingly dark. The latter is especially true of the middle-life woman who recognizes ''lost time'' in expressing her creativity, achieving her career goals, and/or forming trusting relationships with men and starting a family of her own. The implicit or explicit challenge such a woman brings is ''Who cares? Why care?'' and she can present a very convincing case for feeling this way. In the area of her presenting problem, she is convinced of her helplessness and of the unpredictable anxieties of her particular life circumstances.

The diagnostic classifications which typify women entering therapy at this stage are the neurotic disorders such as obsessive–compulsive personality, hysterical personality, and dysthymic disorders. These are the categories which epitomize the social results of strict adherence to traditional female role specializations. The ideals of passive dependency and restricted competence fit well with ongoing projections of heroism onto men and male authorities.

In terms of competence assessment, these women have usually achieved a great deal in their lives although they disclaim most of it. They may have amassed educational accomplishments, reared children, managed households, become cultured in literature and the arts, and learned many complex skills of ordinary living (e.g., baking, cooking, sewing, etc.); but there is usually a substantial gap between their adaptive mastery of actual skills/knowledge and the competence they will recognize in themselves. It is important that competence is not confused with critical judgment, however. Psyche women are typically rather judgmental about their own areas of mastery and accomplishment although they do not openly claim authority. The paradoxical nature of their disclaimed authority may come out in critical judgments of the therapist's or others' skills and knowledge, and in double-bind statements (e.g., "You can go ahead and try to help me, but I don't think it will work.").

Typical environmental stresses are financial and relational. Older and middle-aged women may be unable to support themselves financially. Whether they live alone, with grown children, or with their husbands, such women encounter relational difficulties when they are convinced that their female power has diminished with the passing years. Friends and relatives retreat from the woman who is dedicated to convincing others that she has declined in power (e.g., attractiveness to men) and personal authority.

Younger women entering therapy at this stage tend to suffer from similar stresses without the obvious vulnerability to depression. Unmarried or married women in their mid-20s to late 30s hover between two beliefs: They will be saved by marriage and a family, or they will be doomed by marriage and a family. They may reluctantly acknowledge their contributions and competences in a career or interpersonal realm, but somehow they do not feel they are "good enough." If they have not lived out "ideals" of marriage and childrearing, they believe these activities would compensate for the lack of self-worth they feel. If they have not lived out career or creative ideals, they believe that these would bring them self-esteem. Younger women may not speak openly of their basic sense of dissatisfaction with self at the outset of therapy, and they may even question the ideals they secretly hold for themselves, but they will eventually reveal that they assume the promise of a more "secure" life lies in what they "have yet to do." In other words, they evaluate themselves and their acquired skills and knowledge through a lens of deficit thinking: The best possibilities for satisfaction lie in what yet must be accomplished (i.e., where they have chosen "wrongly").

The limitations of the traditional roles of wife and mother are dramatically expressed in the dreams and preoccupations of women at the heroic stage of animus development. The following dream is from Maude, whose earlier dream of *Mission Impossible* was related in Chapter 5. This dream occurred more than 3 years into her therapy, almost 2 years after the earlier dream. She was struggling to establish herself in a caregiving profession commonly identified with women, about which she held many traditional masculine misgivings. Maude consciously acknowledged her struggle to value her interests and activities, which contributed both to her material well-being and to a sense of satisfaction in her marital relationship. Still she was troubled constantly that her work in an allied health field was "unscientific" and was not as good as the work done by professionals who had completed medical school. Her dream depicts her imprisonment by a severely judgmental, critical animus complex. He is represented by the male doctor, her own heroic ideal of the moment.

There is an old woman locked up in an asylum. The room has been locked for a long time and the women was kept in the locked closet within. She wanted out, but was being held prisoner. Her husband came to get her and had gotten into her room without permission. He had some plan to free her, but the male doctor was really shocked that the husband loved her so much, that he was going to save her. This room is in the basement. The old woman had thought the place was a hotel when she came, but then she had not been strong enough to leave. I watched all of this and didn't think the husband knew what was going on, and I was afraid the doctor would lock both of them up. But it was clear at the end that the husband would get the old woman out. I thought to myself, "The husband might be a little crazy too," and concluded, "I don't know because it's hard to tell who's crazy and who's not."

The dream hardly needs commentary. The image of the old woman locked in the closet of a prison, a prison she had assumed was a hotel, is clearly expressive of what women rightfully fear in the traditional role of dependent wife. Maude had spent her adolescent years fearing that she was crazy, especially because of a variety of troubles she was having with her father (see Chap. 5). Her marriage to a man quite opposite in style from her father was developing into a rich and supportive companionship as Maude's therapy proceeded. As a result of her own confrontation with depression, Maude was beginning to question many of the categories for "crazy" as she had applied them to women. Her new insight into the male-dominant aspects of labeling the "mentally ill" comes through in her humorous observation at the end of the dream. Maude gradually developed a more ironic, humorous stance in relationship to her critical heroic animus.

The actual alienation of many older women from positions of power, and even from relationships with men, is frightening to younger women as they anticipate aging. It is extremely depressing to older women. A woman identified with the negative Mother (Venus) can become bitter with jealousy and resentment toward younger women. She displaces her anger at the patriarchy onto the Pandora images that younger women often represent in our society. She covets the powers of younger women as they appear from the masculine perspective, but she feels herself locked into a prison of passive dependency on men.

Bitterness, envy, and poisonous aggression can disrupt the therapeutic alliance between an older client and younger woman therapist at the Psyche stage of animus development. When the younger woman attempts to analyze the client's projections (onto men) of self-reliance, creativity, and emotional security, the client may respond with aggressive challenges (sometimes labeled "narcissistic defenses"). Like Venus, she will set one test after another, and if the therapist fails, the client will feel a triumph of her own depression. The therapist must be other than simply heroically rational and analytical in response to such a client's aggressive challenge. Instead of responding by "outdoing" the client's rational explanations of her resignation to bitterness, the therapist will be more effective in allying herself with the Mother complex (the complaints of Venus). By empathic understanding of the realistic limitations of female power and authority in a patriarchal culture, the therapist can gradually guide the client to internalize elements of her heroic animus complex.

In the face of a lifetime of lost opportunities for mastery and competence, the older woman is vulnerable to an increased sense of helplessness if she is urged to take on tasks that she believes are too difficult for her. Often the therapist and client are confused about how the woman can actually increase her sense of competence; typically, it is best to increase the client's empowerment in activities over which she already experiences mastery.

A 49-year-old client, Connie, entered therapy because she was concerned about her lack of enthusiasm for further pursuing her artistic work, though she had had considerable success at it. She was a weaver and had been acclaimed for the shows and classes she had put together in the previous 5 years. Connie had practiced her art "on the side" over the 15 years she had reared a family of seven children, supported her husband's career, and managed a household. When she entered therapy she had been divorced for 5 years, during which time she had been the primary parent to four teenagers, three of whom were still living at home. She was bitter about her husband's departure and remarriage. She experienced it as a desertion and she was not hopeful about pursuing other long-term relationships with men.

She and her younger therapist had frequent therapeutic misalliances in which the younger woman tended to idealize the accomplishments and creative capacity of the older client. The therapist saw in her client possibilities for heroic development, in both her artistic and relational life, that the client was reluctant and even resistant to claim. Consequently, Connie often feared the "rejection" of her therapist for not "achieving what the therapist seemed to want"—that is, an increased sense of competence and mastery in her achievements. Connie tended to focus her anger on the therapist, who could "do anything she wanted with her life." The client projected the heroic animus onto the therapist and then responded as the bitter Venus, in challenging attacks, or as the passive Psyche, expecting supporting nurturance. Here is a dream of Connie's which occurred about 4 months into therapy:

I am pulling my 21-year-old son in a large wagon over a rutted, bumpy path
through a wood . . . not a dense wood. We can see a house down the valley
on our left. We are looking for a place for my son to camp. The rest of us had
arranged to stay in the house, but my son has come unexpectedly and so has
to sleep out. As I pull him along, there are protruding tree roots, an old car-
riage stuck in dry mud, making our path rather hazardous. The wagon finally
tips over and my son shoots down an embankment at a great speed. I look on
in horror thinking that he will break his leg, but he stands right up when he
reaches the bottom so I know he is O.K. The place where he slid down is like
a hard, polished clay slide. As I look down I see a family of four crossing a
stream and drying their feet. To the right of them is a pond and I notice a
woman's body floating face up on the water. She is fully clothed and I think
she is dead, but then I noticed that her mouth is moving slightly. I watch her
very intently from the top of the embankment and can just make out that she
is swimming very slowly with hardly any movement. I think that my son will
not want to camp out there.

The alliance between the heroic animus (son) and the Mother complex
(being pulled by Mother in a wagon) is a common theme at this stage.
Her depression can be understood as the weight of her own potential
development (expressed also in her waking relationship with this son)
when it is projected onto others and denied in herself. At the Conscientious Stage of ego development, Connie was often exhausted by her
perfectionism—an unending series of self-criticisms and an unwillingness to attempt anything that could not be done perfectly well. Her
depression about failure and lost possibilities was her current experience of the death marriage to a "perfect hero." In her family life, this
woman was vulnerable to arguing with her children over their identity
issues which arose, in part, in her own unrealized animus potential.

    The consequences of the death marriage show up most poignant-
ly in dream images of the old Mother—and in bitter complaints—in
women of all ages. Feelings of stagnation and resentment, usually mis-
directed at oneself for having made the "wrong choices" or having
missed the opportunities at hand, are the primary motifs of the old
Mother. When the woman is consciously identified with the Mother
complex in this form, her unconscious preoccupations will take the
form of the heroic animus. Depending on her relationships with men
in waking life, the woman may be able to rely on the complex to "carry
her through" when she needs an aggressive or agentive response.
When working in her favor, she may be able to speak or act in ways
that are surprisingly courageous, even to her. When it is not working
in her favor, however, the complex tends to be experienced as a "drag"
or subtle ongoing irritation with her life circumstances—an irritating
reminder of the growth that she feels incapable of making.

    The following dream illustrates Linda's response to her negative

Mother complex. Linda is the 46-year-old professional woman who had the dream of bringing the youthful animus "punk" into the light, earlier in the chapter. The following dream occurred about the same time in her therapy when Linda was actively struggling to withdraw her heroic projections (onto valued men in her life) and to feel herself worthy of partnership.

I was first at a sorority house and didn't feel well. [In fact, she was ill with a virus at the time of this dream.] There seemed to be six different containers of flowers in a circle; it was lovely. Someone gave me some flowers.

Some woman, blond, older, and very attractive, came in and talked about this wonderful energy within her. She spread apart her legs and it had something to do with finding the energy within.

Then I went to Mother's house. She and Dad were there. It was her house but it was white and cold. She was furious with me. I was lying on the floor, not feeling well, in a fur coat. She said what a mess I was and how I was in the midst of having a nervous breakdown. I said I was not and "You're the one who has had a nervous breakdown." Then I went upstairs and told her I did not want to talk to her again for a while as I was so angry with her. I knew there would be trouble. Later she said "Well, we are going to talk, aren't we?" I think we were sitting down to dinner and I did not answer her. A friend of mine came in, at that moment, and I just raised my eyebrows at her.

During the discovery of the heroic animus and its integration into the woman's sense of self, we have noticed the intrapsychic arousal of the negative Mother complex, even in women who have felt free of its consequences for some years. It is as though the old Mother is challenged by the self-determination of her Daughter, as though this psychic marriage to one's own heroism were a challenge to the position of the Mother complex in the woman's personality. It seems to us that as long as the heroic animus is projected and denied, the hold of the Mother on the personality of the woman is still very powerful. It is as though the attitude of the negative Mother—that the woman is presumed to be small, dependent, and weak—keeps a strong hold until the woman embraces her own heroism.

Because the client may have identified her actual mother with the negative Mother complex, it is critical that the therapist emphasize the concept of "complex," as an internalized cluster of associations and feelings around an archetypal core, and distinguish this aspect of the client's personality from the actual mother. Whether young or old, the female client depends to some extent on cherishing her actual mother to revitalize her own female authority. The client's self-esteem is enhanced by separating in her awareness the effect of a complex that derives from early childhood experiences and is infused with emotional arousal, and the characteristics of a "woman like your mother." Be-

ing able to see both the strengths and weaknesses in her actual mother—and valuing the strengths—prepares the client to take on her own
tasks of mastery.

Let us look briefly at the typical phases of the therapeutic relationship with a Psyche woman, having sketched out the early phase in
some detail.

Differentiation of the Animus Complex
and the Negative Mother Complex

This first phase establishes an analytical relationship between client and
therapist regarding the effects of the animus complex on the client's
personality. Through interpretation, clarification, and use of empathic
rapport, the client confronts the meaning of her heroic animus as it has
been projected, unconsciously identified with, and denied. Interpretations of the therapeutic relationship, and of both early and ongoing relationships with men, are the foci of this phase. Dream interpretations
are useful, not only for defining personal and archetypal meanings, but
for motivating the client to claim the dimensions of her own animus
complex as well. The negative Mother complex can be distinguished
clearly from the client's own identity, especially in its effects on her
motivation for change and mastery.

In the therapist's encounter with the client's anger and aggression,
maintaining a firm empathy and interpreting distorted or displaced aggression will assist the client in recognizing and integrating her motives. Encouraging the client to take responsibility for temporary,
nonrational feelings is essential. This responsibility demands that the
client make a choice about whether or not she desires to express these
feelings. Taking responsibility for feelings should include the client's
recognition that transitory feelings are not a part of her identity (e.g.,
"I *am* depressed" is identification of oneself with a mood).

Integrating the Heroic Animus

When the characteristics of the client's own heroism—desire for greater
mastery and competence—are understood, then the therapist supports
her integration of the complex. Through new learning, work, therapeutic homework, etc., the client tries out new activities and attitudes,
which permit greater courage, creativity, and enthusiasm in her daily
life. By and large, these activities are tried outside of the therapeutic
session, but they are reported within it. The therapist helps the client
monitor any continuing problems with internalized inferiority, perfectionism, and self-effacement.

Understanding Personal Responsibility

The final phase in the treatment of the Psyche woman, which is typically brief, involves making closure on matters of responsibility in this woman's current life. Differentiating between "happenings" and "agency" (Schafer, 1978) is the crux of this matter. The client must fully understand that she is personally responsible for matters that are within her conscious control: certain circumstances of her life and her own attitude. Responsibility for tragedies of the past, for illness and for other unpredictable accidents of life needs to be rationally disclaimed. At the same time, the matter of personal choice (i.e., "What do you *want* to do about this?") is constantly emphasized as legitimate "agency" in setting a direction in her life, no matter what the circumstances. It is essential in this final stage that the limitations of human consciousness and the inevitability of inner conflict be recognized by the client as continuing parts of human life, no matter how masterful or aware she becomes.

The final two phases of therapy with the Psyche woman are marked by a strong collaborative relationship between client and therapist, who are able to share a symbolic reality. In fact, the second and third phases are so pleasantly mutual and dynamically creative that the therapist must continuously assess her/his own need to keep the client in therapy.

We have discovered that Psyche clients in the second and third phases of treatment often provide us with rich insights about their own dilemmas. The client's dreams and the therapist's motivations to continue sessions should be carefully monitored for signs of the approaching end of therapy. When the client can interpret her own dreams in a substantially accurate way, when dream images point to the end of therapy, and when the therapist *too* enthusiastically anticipates this client's session, the close of treatment is coming into view.

Let us go back to the second phase of the treatment process and look at some examples from actual cases. An unconscious embrace of the heroic animus often happens quite naturally when a woman falls in love and marries, enters a new creative endeavor, or makes a new contract with someone she admires. Maude, the 26-year-old client in her third year of therapy, had the following dream. Her animus is imaged as her husband, a "feminine" man in comparison to her father. Her early adult adaptation had been as a Father's Daughter and she had entered therapy in the Pandora stage of animus development. In the first several years of her marriage, Maude had distrusted her husband and often simply refused to listen to his advice, or secretly belittled his style and manner. From the standpoint of her authoritarian Father complex, she had seen her husband as "only a boy." At the time of this dream, Maude was reviewing her husband and saw him now as a competent, creative, and exciting alternative to her Father complex. She and her husband were having a renewal of romance as Maude was becoming more confident of her own worth. The following dream depicts both the embrace and the confrontation with the old Mother.

I have taken my lover (now my husband) away from another woman. I kiss him passionately. He doesn't look quite himself; he is taller and more handsome, very handsome. When we kiss, he lifts me off the ground. He feels so strong. This embrace seems awe-inspiring to the crowd watching. Just before he and I leave together, my old aunt takes off her wig and exposes her matted hair underneath. (This seems to be some kind of signal.)

Note the energy and power of the heroic embrace. The inflation (it is awe-inspiring) is balanced by the old aunt removing her wig, showing the consequences of simply identifying with the embrace. If Maude were to remain captured by the embrace itself, the enthusiasm and momentum of the romantic moment with the heroic other, she could lock herself in an arrangement of "being saved" by a man or she might begin to perpetually search for the perfect male companion. Instead, she worked hard to integrate both the satisfaction of her newly achieved competence (in terms of furthering her own self-interests in useful work) and the gains of her newly acquired pleasures with her husband (freeing him from her projected desires for achievements of a traditionally masculine sort).

We also encounter another kind of embrace in the dreams and lives of women at this phase of therapy. They often passionately embrace other women, coming face to face with loving the femaleness of the other. Some women actually do choose to turn to a lesbian relationship in integrating an independent heroism. Others dream of lesbian encounters as sexually stimulating and personally pleasurable. We call this image an "embrace of the woman-self" and connect it to the integration of the heroic animus. The greater part of Psyche's adventure is, afterall, her excited connection to the other women in the story: her sisters and Venus. The following dream is not a unique example of this enlivening female embrace: sexual feelings about one's mother. Many of our clients have similar dreams, but this one stands out for its clarity. Andrea, 33, was a graduate student with two children when she entered therapy. She was discovering her own sexuality in a new marriage to a man onto whom she had projected her heroic animus, but she was troubled by a "driven quality" in her daily life and an overly critical Mother complex. About 3 years into her analysis, she had the following dream:

I am lying beside my mother in bed, in a hotel. My mother complains about never being sexually stimulated and I am concerned about whether or not she has ever experienced orgasm. I realize that my father has not made love to her in years. I decide to help my mother have an orgasm and she seems pleased. I feel excited in my own genitals. She opens her blouse and displays her large old breasts. I am aroused, knowing that I can give her an orgasm, but then I am afraid that she might have dried up, that her vagina may not lubricate. I notice that she doesn't have pubic hair, the result of aging. I stimulate her and find that she lubricates easily and has a very comforting orgasm. She seems to have no problem enjoying sex; I am relieved to find that she is sexually experienced.

Andrea had believed, since childhood, that her mother was not sexually active. Obviously, she had maintained a parentified attitude toward her mother, becoming overly concerned for her mother's safety and well-being. In the dream she is relieved of her guilt about her own sexual pleasure by discovering that the Mother is also sexual and that she has control of this. Andrea's embrace of the Mother was preceded by many dreams of the Mother's anger and even rage. Through the differentiation of the Mother complex from the actual mother, Andrea had come to love and even enjoy her mother in a renewed way, reminiscent of her earlier childhood feelings of admiration and warmth for this woman.

Confrontation with the Underground Goddess—in the form of hidden competence and pleasures—is both a potential loss and a potential regeneration as we have stated. In this phase of integration, the client sometimes experiences herself as being "essentially alone" and wandering around her daily life with only a half-remembered sense of who she is or was. The client needs a great deal of support during this process, because she may grieve the loss of many potentialities in herself. Encounters with lost time, lost child-bearing potential, lost educational opportunities, and lost beauty or youth are common themes.

Depth of insight and reconnection to legitimate anger are the primary goals at this point. The therapist's familiarity with underlying issues of female gender identity, her acquaintance with idealized images of female authority (e.g., goddesses), and her awareness of what constitute realistic aspirations toward new roles for women in a patriarchal society will make a great difference to the outcome of this second phase. Reductive interpretations of analytical material that are too critical of the client's mother (e.g., that she was "overwhelming," "dangerous," or "devouring") can be especially harmful. The client needs the support of some ideal images of female authority to assist her in accomplishing the major changes she needs to make in her attitude and daily life.

Some clients dream of revolutions during this phase. Andrea had the following dream about a year after she dreamed of giving her mother an orgasm.

I live in New York City in a decadent period. There is a lot of street violence. I must leave my hotel room for a job interview, and my husband, who is supposed to protect me, does not show up. Suddenly, I am in the line of fire in some kind of street attack between gangs. Although I know that I am not the target, I am afraid of being killed. I slip under a parked car for protection.

After the firing subsides, a friendly taxi cab driver, who looks a bit like Anthony Quinn in *Zorba*, picks me up. He drives me down a steep hill and we are in my aunt's neighborhood from my childhood, in a Black neighborhood at the bottom of a steep hill.

There has been an accident at the bottom of the hill. At first I see only a Black woman, a housewife dressed in a shirtwaist dress and apron. She is moaning and crying for her husband. I think that he must have been killed in the accident and my heart goes out to her. Then I see that the man's body is still in the street; it is covered by a child's red wagon. Two young children, at about the age of 6 or 7, a boy and a girl, are seated in the wagon. The taxi driver suggests that I look at the Black man, that I remove the wagon from over his face. I do not want to look because I abhor violence and do not want to see any blood or torn flesh. But the driver insists and seems not to respond to my fears. He pulls the wagon off the man's face and I see a young Black man of about 33, who is good-looking and unmarked by the accident, except for a sort of placenta and blood enclosure around his face. I say to myself, "Oh, that's a birth mask." I think that the blood may be from the accident, but I am confused. At that moment, the Black man opens his eyes and smiles. I think to myself: Well, this man isn't dead at all. Maybe he's just been born. The driver replaces the wagon solemnly, and no one says anything.

The confusion between birth and death is another common theme at this phase of integrating the heroic animus. Andrea had actually been involved in a dispute about her job, a situation in which she needed her anger to defend her rights. Her movement out into the street violence and her ability to look directly at this new animus figure are assisted by a guide, an unknown male who is reminiscent of Zorba. Male guide figures of unknown origin (i.e., the "wise old men") often appear in women's dreams during the turmoil of new heroic actions and attitudes.

At this time, also, the therapist may become the target of idealizing projections of a "complete woman." In a sense, the therapist is cast as a new ideal mother, the mentor who is both strong and nurturant. This situation is quite different from the earlier stages of animus development when the therapist was seen as Great Mother or when the therapist was completely confused with the client's more primitive identity images. A well-maintained analytical objectivity (i.e., the analytical frame) in which the client is minimally exposed to the therapist's private life is essential for clarifying the real boundaries of the idealization. Clarification of the distinct potentials of the client are increasingly necessary as the treatment enters its final phase.

A dream of Linda's will illustrate some of the problematic confusions between therapist and client. Linda was involved in new creative projects and in changing her life-style to allow herself more freedom for creative expression. Using an internalized ideal image of her therapist to strengthen her courage (e.g., asking herself "What would my therapist say?" in moments of turmoil), Linda had proceeded to develop new arrangements in her work schedule and daily life.

I married a man (who looked like the husband of a valued woman friend) who was a psychologist. I was not very happy because I hardly knew him. We had Thanksgiving dinner, and earlier that day I had been thinking about how unhappy I was and how I didn't really know how I had gotten myself into all this.

We all danced together and got ready for a party. His mother came over and I was sort of quiet and withdrawn. Then suddenly he said he had to leave for the church service and would be back around an hour and a half from then. I felt awful that we had not known he would leave because we hadn't eaten. I decided we'd put the meal out on the kitchen table and people could serve themselves and go to the living room. I went through his apartment and saw all this lovely china. I think it was gold and orange and cream. But I wanted my own china. I noticed he had collected a lot.

Then my therapist and I were in this wonderful room alone. It had a huge glass window. Suddenly the room started to pitch around and I realized that it was a houseboat. We leaned way over near the water and I was afraid the glass would break and we would fall into the water. It just kept pitching, though, and we were getting gorgeous sights of towers and ships. Suddenly we saw a whole series of Chinese boats. If we hadn't been so frightened, we really would have loved it. (I'm not sure my therapist was frightened.)

Then somehow we were on the shore. We were looking at shops. There was a little bridal shop and we went in. I asked if there were any bridesmaids' pictures. One picture seemed to be of my therapist getting married, in a lovely long white dress. Then she put on some mascara and looked exotic.

The dream depicts a marriage to the "wrong" heroic animus, to a psychologist like her therapist. Later the dream produces the therapist's wedding picture! From this dream, the client and therapist were able to clarify the client's fears of disappointing her therapist. Linda worried that she was not changing her life-style "fast enough to suit you." Differentiating the mentor relationship with the friend in Linda's profession (in the dream) from the therapeutic relationship, focusing on Linda's own resources and current stresses, and examining the therapist's idealized projections onto Linda, all contributed to making a more realistic plan for the client's life changes.

The final phase of therapy with the Psyche woman must include a recognition of the universality of inner conflict and the meaning of personal responsibility. There is no standard way in which these can be expressed through case illustrations because they vary from person to person. We have chosen a dream from a client in her mid-60s, however, who was courageously reexamining her own heroic potential. At the Autonomous Stage of ego development, Diane came to therapy in order to further her creative interests in writing. She had been painting and lecturing throughout many years of her adult life, even as she had been rearing five children and supporting her husband's career. Most of her early adulthood had been spent in the Pandora stage, with her animus projected (in the form of the Father complex) onto her articulate and well-educated husband. Over the years, Diane had come to claim many of her own competences and rational strengths, but she was not secure in these. Furthermore, in establishing these she had grown distant and angry with her husband. She wanted very much to repair her relationship with him in their final years together. The following dream occurred in her third therapy session. She was already poised to integrate her heroic animus and quickly made progress.

I am at a party at some friends' house on a lake. I see a pathetic couple from the university. They are a mother and daughter. They have decorated themselves very attractively, but I know this is partly to hide how depressed they feel. The daughter is overeager, the ''soft'' type that I despise, and her mother can't let her do a thing alone. They are tied together like twin sufferers. If this is what happens to mothers and daughters, I am better off for not having a mother!

Later I am with my daughter-in-law and her little boy. He is so adorable: wicked, full of energy, and itching for mischief. He comes up next to a Big Bear Man at the party and goes to sleep in his arms. This man, unknown to me, is a male type that I am always looking for—relaxed, accepting, loving, quiet, nonverbal. Big thing is his solid rock quality. He is *there*, to be depended upon, sprawled upon. You can go to sleep in his lap, and even active little boys, like my grandson, are soothed by his charm. With this Big Bear Man, I could survive, live.

I tell him what a beautiful thing it is to see my grandson fall asleep in his arms, really just sprawled across the man's lap. The man just sits there, neither encouraging nor rejecting the child, just *being*. Brings a great sense of warmth and peace.

The recognition of the Big Bear Man as her own heroic animus was a liberating awareness for Diane, opening up a new perspective on her creative work and her relationship with her husband. Although Diane had had much Jungian analysis in the past and had been aware of the concept of "animus" and its traditional meaning as inferior objectivity in women, she had not understood her own relationship to the complex. Through interpreting this dream and following through on many of the ideas it awakened in her, Diane was able to withdraw this projection (onto her husband)—and with it some of her unfair anger toward him for being the man he was—and to come to terms with her Mother complex, especially with her identification with the positive Great Mother side. The dream displays a pathetic mother–daughter pair. This, Diane understood to be herself bound to an overly nurturant orientation in her relationships with others, including her husband. The nurturant imperative that she often unconsciously assumed had resulted in resentment and in feelings of abandonment. She would care for others—whether they wanted it or not—because she felt so unprotected or undernurtured herself.

At the same time, this dream brought to light the idea of loss in terms of its irreparable effects. Diane's mother had died just after Diane's birth. Losing her mother so early had had major consequences for her overall personality development, but these had not been merely deficits. The observation in the dream that she is "better off for not having a mother" was especially important to Diane, who began to claim some of the benefits of this early separation. And yet the separation also led to an ongoing desire to be nurtured and contained, held by the Big Bear Man. Since the bear is central to Great Mother symbolism, we were able to draw connections between her heroic complex and her positive Mother complex. Acceptance of both the positive and negative aspects of the loss of her mother was the framework for Diane's recognition of the effects of inner conflict on her personality and life.

Over the next several months, Diane began to write creatively about her experience as a mother, in regard to her own Mother complex and in regard to the loss of her mother. Eventually she published a paper in a professional journal which related her experiences to a cycle of mythic stories. Diane began to live out the benefits of her inner conflict between the heroic animus and the Mother complex, neither giving in to despair nor to idealizing (of the Big Bear Man) in her relationship with the men in her life. As a consequence of this creative development, Diane entered a new partnership with her husband, whom she no longer resented for not providing the Big Bear quality of relationship she had desired. Similarly, she found that her envy of her husband's intellectual achievements diminished considerably as she accrued achievements of her own.

The completion of this stage, whether through therapy or life development, is signaled by the end of embittered servitude and envy. As women value their own contributions, choose selectively (in their own self-interest) how and when they desire to provide for others, and live out some kind of imaginative expression in work, they enter a new partnership with animus. It is as though they have available to themselves new vitality and resources never before experienced. This sense of partnership with one's own creative process and freedom from internalized inferiority mark the beginning of the next stage.

8

Stages Four and Five: Restoration of Authority

The fourth stage of animus development involves a clear, conscious confrontation with the oppressive conditions of women in a patriarchal society. Becoming aware of these monstrous conditions, which have been accepted and rationalized for women, is analogous to Ariadne's confrontation with the minotaur, the monstrous underground product of her mother's rage. This stage culminates with a woman making an active choice in favor of her own self-interest and self-fulfillment. By learning to reflect upon herself and her cultural context objectively, she recognizes the symbolic connection between her own personality and her tribe (other women), and between her own consciousness and the heroic animus complex, which she has unconsciously fashioned in a patriarchal society. Through the connection to her masculine heroism, she discovers that she is the source of her own worthiness and the foundation of her own authority.

Claiming personal authority and consciously acknowledging the importance of cherished relationships are the major psychological tasks of this stage. When a woman has integrated both, she will have achieved the reliable integration of her animus as Partner Within. Her masculine complex is a part of her conscious personality. Prerequisites for entering this fourth stage are a heightened awareness of individuality, an appreciation of inner conflict, and an ability to sustain a symbolic inner dialogue with oneself through dreams and creative expression.

To understand the confrontation that takes place between women at this stage and the oppressive conditions of the culture, it is first necessary to understand the paradoxical nature of motherhood. The ideals of compassion, for example, can be credited to the way in which women are socialized to be mothers. Care, sustenance, dependence, and empathy are the worthy aspects of female socialization that mark us as unique in our gender-associated behaviors. On the other hand, servility, passivity, inferiority, and low self-esteem plague all of us whose contributions to society are continuously devalued. Repeatedly, we find ourselves in the impossible situation of having the responsibility for the sustenance of others while we have no corresponding power. When we face this condition and understand the way in which it has been frozen within our own fears and self-denigrations, we recognize larger social and cultural issues that demand a broader perspective. This is the perspective of female authority and objective empathy. Dally (1982) speaks from such a perspective in her historical account of motherhood. Both objective and empathic, Dally is an example of a woman whose heroic animus is consciously integrated. For example:

> Mothers bear the burden not only as child-rearers but also as scape-goats. Their role [has] become increasingly uncertain and untenable. The needs of young children are increasingly at variance with the organization and way of life of our society, and this gap is filled partly by idealizing the mother and partly by denigrating and humiliating her. The situation is frozen by making it extremely difficult for her to see the situation realistically and so she is unable to do anything about it. (p. 18)

Seeing one's situation realistically and doing something about it are the hallmarks of later animus development, that is, of the woman who has internalized the animus complex as heroic Partner Within. She achieves a new freedom whereby she can better adapt to the competing roles that are necessarily a part of her daily life. She gets better at managing stress and compensating for vulnerabilities through her increased awareness of and confidence in herself. She also has a sense of increased responsibility, claimed partly through a recognition that she has *constructed* her own experience throughout her lifetime, and partly through claiming her authority to state her own truths. Such a woman does not disclaim her shameful, doubting, aggressive, or rageful impulses; but she can put them in context so that she is neither overwhelmed nor excessively defended. A woman at this stage, then, clearly grows beyond her identification with Mother, but she does not leave behind the issue of motherhood. Rather, she integrates an understanding of motherhood into a larger social context.

The completion of this fourth stage of animus development is evident when a women has developed a more or less reliable ability to discriminate between her own authority and others' (especially men's) reality: She takes others' anxieties and criticisms less personally and resists hearing passing remarks as serious commentary on her identity. She feels freer to love the activities in which she is engaged, from relational caring to creative work. Her identity is no longer bound to the inferior status of female gender nor to the confinement of a particular role, such as wife or mother. Consequently she is less anxious.

The major struggle continuing to develop throughout and beyond this stage is the striving for personal authority across diverse roles. Consciously acknowledging that her identity attitudes and attributes are complex and in conflict, a woman must realize that she cannot perform all roles equally well. She must give up perfectionism once and for all. In evaluating herself in relation to other women, she has become aware of her realistic competences and vulnerabilities.

When she is vulnerable to feeling inadequate, she seeks additional support and arranges to get help. Getting help with housework, child-care, administrative tasks, or even with pumping gas is a manner of being strong when one knows oneself. Arranging her interpersonal and physical environment to support her self-esteem and pleasure, a woman at this stage renounces the unattainable and stops trying to be all things to all people. The fantasy of overaccommodation, part of the patriarchal ideal of motherhood, presupposes that there are no boundaries between oneself and others, so that one is constantly available to meet others' needs. It is for this very psychological state that many women are blamed when they are called "overprotective" or "self-effacing."

Women at this stage value the satisfaction they attain in diverse roles. Openly claiming the pleasures of doing housework, of earning one's own income, and of expressing oneself articulately are examples of ways in which these women manifest satisfactions. Such enthusiasm can be felt even in the midst of loss and suffering. Recognition of what has not been attained or what one has had to set aside does not prevent a sense of gratitude for current well-being. This kind of belief in her own goodness permits the woman to be genuinely interested in the development of others.

What kinds of women tend to attain this stage of animus development? Because we have only our clinical observations as data (and so few clients come to us at this stage), we have turned to larger studies to understand how women go on developing throughout adulthood. A study reported by Baruch et al. (1983)—involving about 300 American women in the 35 to 50 age span (data collected from 1979 to 1980)—provides some clear indications. Throughout their book (*Life Prints*; Baruch et al., 1983), the authors stress the important contribution made by paid work, especially challenging work, to a sense of well-being in middle-aged women. What is most surprising, perhaps, is that, overall, the authors discovered that the busiest (and hence potentially most conflicted) women were most satisfied with their lives. For example:

> A key finding of our study . . . is that the women who scored highest on all the indices of well-being were married women with children

who have high-prestige jobs. This is the group one would expect to be the most harried, rushed, and conflicted—and yet they seem to come through with flying colors. This finding dovetails with that of a major study of psychiatric disorder reported in 1977 by Frederic W. Ilfeld. . . . The researchers surveyed 2,299 Chicago households, and found that the percentage of women with "high symptomatology"— a lot of problems—was twice that of men's. The only group of women who had symptom rates as low as men were employed women whose occupational status was high. (p. 143)

The combination of intimate relationships with children and partners and satisfying work, which is rewarded by status and pay, seems to predict the greatest possibility for development. Of course, this kind of life-style by no means elminates stress or distress. But with a variety of activities and sources of support available, a woman has many places on which to lean for self-esteem. When she is feeling low about her work, she can remember her pleasure in relationships. Conversely, she can congratulate herself on earning a good income when she feels lousy about her mothering. The more sources of support and peer-recognized competence available to a woman, the more likely she will be to integrate a sense of personal authority with the limitations to perfection she has come to identify.

By contrast, women who have a difficult time reaching the later stages of animus development in adulthood are often those who have chosen the exclusive roles of wife or mother, as society has dictated to them through promise of happiness based upon material dependence. According to Baruch *et al.* (1983):

> By midlife, as we saw, role strain—feeling pulled apart, over-loaded—is more a problem for mothers at home than for women in the workforce. Employment seems to help a woman to cope with stress, while being responsible for raising children may be today's high-risk job. (p. 248)

Confronting the social meanings of the institutions of marriage and motherhood in a patriarchal society arouses a fear of "abandonment" in many women, especially older women. All that is implied by the concept of identity confusion—anxiety, paranoia, loss of self, loss of agency, etc.—is part of the experience of seeing the paradoxical nature of female gender identity. Consequently, this kind of deeper apprehension of the meaning of her gender will be quite threatening to a woman and should not be foisted on her prematurely, that is, before she has secured the possibility of a variety of life choices. Many women never arrive at this point. As we stressed earlier, this fourth stage of animus development remains a rare achievement among adult women. The cognitive complexity (beyond formal thought operations), interpersonal maturity, and symbolic acumen required for integrating the animus complex entirely into self-awareness are the products of privilege for women in our society. Until we have changed social conditions of the lives of many, these prerequisites for a securely conscious masculinity will belong to the lucky and the few.

ABANDONMENT AND THE PARTNER WITHIN

The theme of abandonment emerges and reemerges in women's development as they come to terms repeatedly with the realistic dimensions of dependence in their lives. At this stage, abandonment is a symbolic theme of inner conflict, usually experienced as a fear that one's knowledge, authority, or skill will suddenly disappear in the midst of a crisis. A woman fears that she cannot make it through her own creative and autonomous tasks without some shameful or even disastrous consequence. In other words, the woman fears she will be abandoned by her heroic animus complex, as it is not securely integrated into consciousness and may seem to come and go at will.

A women entering this fourth stage has already consciously differentiated emotional and material dependence. She is aware of the distinction between psychological independence and merely living alone, although she may have to be reminded. Such a woman cherishes relationships that have sustained her and remembers that these other people are also independent adults responsible for their own lives. Occasionally, though, such a woman confuses her fear of abandonment by her inner resources with a fear of being abandoned by her partner. Fears of betrayal and jealousies involving female competitors are still problematic from time to time, although a woman will usually be able to recognize immediately the folly of such preoccupations. She may also occasionally project her heroic animus onto a man, but this also is rarer and more easily understood.

If a woman enters this stage but does not complete it, she may remain rather literal minded about moral issues linked to commitment, duty, responsibility, and difference. In other words, she may devote herself too literally to changing others and to moving the society in general toward achieving the conditions of human freedom without an adequate concern for her own self-interest. Consequently, she will become embittered, depressed, burnt out, and angry about a fight which she feels is perpetual and ungratifying. Such a woman does not manifest pleasure or satisfaction in her daily life, the kind of satisfaction that frees her from envy and jealousy. When a woman feels generally secure in having her own perspective, intrinsic to and formed out of her experience, she will be able to sustain inner strength. Without this attitude, a woman even at this stage is vulnerable to periodic severe depressions and impulsive expression of aggression related to the rage she feels about her personal and cultural conditions.

ARIADNE AND THESEUS

We have chosen the story of Ariadne and Theseus to depict the major emotional themes of this stage. The story is suitable, although not entirely adequate, because it portrays female heroism in the context of partiarchal culture. We interpret the minotaur to be the monstrous by-product of the buried matriarchal societies (i.e., the bull, with its crescent horns as an image of the moon, is strongly associated with matriarchal deities prior to the Greeks). Ariadne enters the underground labyrinth of the minotaur's home with a fearless confidence in her own awareness and intuition. Several versions of her story are extant. We recount the following details in our own summary retold (not quoted) from Kerenyi (1974, pp. 269–272).

> Ariadne is the daughter of King Minos and Queen Pasiphae. Pasiphae is sometimes called the daughter of the moon, sometimes of the sun. Pasiphae mated with a great white bull, in a fit of rage, to produce the monstrous minotaur, the brother of Ariadne. The minotaur plagued the people of Crete (from his habitation in Knossos) for many years, requiring sacrifices of Athenian youths and maidens every nine years. Finally, the hero Theseus comes to Crete from Athens with a special mission to slay this monster and save the people of Crete.
>
> The minotaur inhabits an elaborate labyrinth which had been constructed by Daedalus. Theseus is unsure about how he will find his way out of this intricate maze. Ariadne, a mortal woman, volunteers to accompany him in slaying her own brother in order to save the people of Crete.
>
> In the best-known later versions of the story, Ariadne rescues Theseus through her cleverness. She saves the hero and the children of Athens (sacrificed into the labyrinth) by giving Theseus a thread to guide his way out. In lesser-known earlier versions, Ariadne accompanies Theseus directly into the labyrinth and leads out the hero and the youths by the light of a bejewelled, golden wreath which crowns her head. This wreath, according to these earlier accounts, was given her by Dionysus. Also in these earlier versions, the labyrinth is a spiral from which one can exit safely only after reaching the center.
>
> After the completion of the heroic deed, Ariadne and Theseus sail off for Athens. Theseus abandons his companion on the island

Dia (now called Naxos). She is left there in a swoon, perhaps even dead. She is suddenly awakened, however, by Dionysus, who appears before her in his chariot and takes her as his bride. In one pictorial representation of this moment, Adriadne is ascending to heaven in a chariot very much like that in which Persephone was carried off to the Underworld.

A later story recounts Dionysus's wedding to Ariadne and her transformation into a goddess. Her famous golden wreath is set in the heavens as a constellation, the Crown of Ariadne.

According to Kerenyi (p. 269), the name *Ariadne* was originally spelled *Ariagne* and means "holy" or "pure." Ironically, as he points out, the name is a superlative form of *Hagne*, or Queen of the Underworld, the later title of Persephone. We had not known of the relationship between Persephone and Ariadne when we chose these stories to represent our stages. We have learned to appreciate the connection between the descent to the Underworld and the retrieval of female authority. We wholeheartedly believe that women must confront, and integrate, the hidden meanings and darkness of their femaleness in order to be confident in their experience and values as authentic individuals. Ariadne makes her journey consciously and courageously, different from Psyche's reluctant and less conscious adventure.

We interpret the image of Ariadne as a form of authority that unites consciousness and the complexes. She is an image of a *transcendent function* (in Jungian terminology) that mediates the dialectial relationship between the personal and the archetypal, uniting the mortal with the divine, and rational heroism with underground intuition. Her image suggests a psychological androgyny. In terms of the story, of course, she weds Dionysus—androgynous god and underground hero.

While this story does not give a complete picture of the process of attaining a partnership within, it points to some important aspects of the process. Identity states that may be projected or identified with are those of Ariadne, Theseus, and Dionysus. Typically the woman of this stage will identify with the Ariadne orientation, assuming a poised confidence about coming and going, and about investigating unconscious meaning. She experiences herself as able to encounter unconscious impulses, wishes, fears, and complexes with some certainty of understanding them. She can work freely back and forth between the irrational and the rational.

Theseus, as an image of the animus complex at this stage, is a more developed hero than Eros was. He seems to represent a compassionate rationality and courage. He can, however, abandon the woman at the outreaches of culture, on an obscure island far from home. Ariadne's "thread" can be interpreted as the connecting link between heroic animus and female consciousness under conditions of peril. Such a connection must be maintained in order for the women to return safely to consciousness and ordinary reality when she is coming to terms with the hidden meanings of her life situation and the backstage power arrangements of the patriarchy.

The Dionysian animus is yet another kind of animus complex at this stage of development. As Zeus and Hephaestus were typical animus configurations for the Pandora woman, Theseus and Dionysus form a continuum between rational and nonrational masculinity for the Ariadne woman. A passionate, intoxicating form of masculinity can be projected or internalized by Ariadne women. Popular images of the Dionysian woman currently abound among rock groups and fashion models. The ideal of the Dionysian woman seems more prominent in fashion magazines than in feminist handbooks. A passionately androgynous woman—seductively masculine, commanding, but still womanly—has captured popular imagination in this period. When a woman identifies with a Dionysian animus, she feels intoxicated with power and excited by her masculine possibilities. Often she feels more confident, less inhibited, and more sexual. When she projects this form of the animus, she is vulnerable to being captivated by a man's imagination and compassion for women. This form of animus is distinctly different from the Hephaestian form, which is far cruder, more bound to primitive defenses, awkward, and enraged. Still, however, Dionysian moods and enactments can be troubling for women in this stage, especially if they include alcohol or other drugs, which ease the tension of conflicting role demands.

Vulnerability to feelings of abandonment becomes a theme when the Ariadne woman with a Dionysian animus recognizes that her fears concern her own ability to maintain a conscious responsibility amidst the effects of aggression, sexuality, envy, and other impulses as she comes to terms with her individuality in a patriarchal context. A woman may experience herself to be much darker or more impenetrable than she had previously thought. Acceptance of the meaning or symbolic value of emotional stress from inner and outer conflict requires a tolerance for paradox and ambiguity that demands great psychological insight.

The story of Ariadne depicts some phases or steps which seem congruent with our therapeutic experience of restoration of female authority. In brief, there is a self-initiated descent into the depths (i.e., a willingness to take on an analytical process in understanding oneself), followed by a confrontation with aggressive and deformed aspects of repressed female power (i.e., recognizing rage and hatred, which have developed within, and their effects on one's actions), and finally a freeing of the personality through a meaningful restoration of an attitude which was lost (i.e., a restoration of vitality, youthful motivation/anticipation, and self-determination). The abandonment of Ariadne is relevant as a social commentary, as well as a psychological one, for liberated women today. The self-initiating woman may be rejected and made to feel that she has been abandoned by a society that tolerates only males in its important decision-making and leadership positions.

The transformation of Ariadne from mortal to goddess symbolizes, for us, a woman's ability to transcend the merely personal or social conditions of her life and to fill out her understanding with archetypal or universal symbolic connections. In our experience with women at this stage (and there have been only a handful), we find that the dream image of a "sacred" or "divine" marriage spontaneously appears at a critical point in therapy when the woman is most stressed. Another prevalent theme is the birth of an extraordinary or divine child who can clearly be distinguished from a human child due to its unusual size, shape, or powers.

It is as though the woman must accept a process of unification in her own personality whether or not she is ready for it. By unifying the feminine and masculine, the compassionate and aggressive, her desires and duties, the woman finally sees herself as an individual.

GOALS, STRATEGIES, AND TECHNIQUES OF THERAPY

Few women enter therapy in this stage. Hypothesizing from the women we have seen and from Loevinger's ego development research on women and girls, we guide ourselves toward the following goals.

1. Recognition on the part of client and therapist that the therapeutic endeavor is a mutual partnership in a shared search for meaning: Because client and therapist are likely to be at the same or similar positions in their respective development (in fact, the client may have surpassed the therapist developmentally), shared desires, difficulties, and discoveries should be integrated consciously so that both client and therapist are wholly aware of their own needs and desires in the therapeutic relationship. While this kind of mutual relationship is a tacit goal at all stages, it must be a prominent part of interpretation at this stage because the therapist is vulnerable to idealizing the client and projecting ideal aspects of the therapist's own development onto the client.

2. Acceptance of inner conflict as the process of development: Again, while this is an ultimate implicit goal at other stages, it is constantly recognized now as part of an increasing responsibility to construct meaning and to build self-respect in both client and therapist. Tolerating the tension of opposites, differences in competing roles and attributes, and the tension of opposing meanings (e.g., conscious and unconscious meanings as equally true) should contribute to the client's

ability to recognize and rely on inner conflict as a natural process of growth without prematurely identifying with either side of the conflict and/or exclusively projecting either side onto the therapist.

3. Ability to express feelings by choice and to take responsibility for a feeling life: The client should come to anticipate a discrepancy between inner reality of feelings and outward appearance, with an understanding that opposite feelings (e.g., love and hate) can be experienced at once. Expression of feelings becomes related to individuality as the client encounters her own need for personal fulfillment, or to satisfaction as distinct from impulse gratification. Recognition of a range of opposing inner states, coupled with an awareness that all of the states are transitory and true, will more and more allow a client to choose actively when she will be receptive to expression and when she will be unreceptive. The effort here is to help the client experience herself as the enactor of her own life rather than as a victim who is passively overtaken by her feelings or complexes as the "truth" of any moment.

4. Recognition of the mutual interdependence of self and other in all human endeavors, beginning with the therapeutic relationship: Consonant with the story we have used to express this stage, various life roles become interchangeable through the process of development. Theseus, the hero, is saved by Ariadne, the victim, who is then apparently abandonned by the hero. But the apparent abandonment is a developmental transformation so that the mortal Ariadne dies in order to become the goddess. A deep acceptance of the interdependence of human life leads to an ability to trust the developmental process and to disperse fears of abandonment.

5. Realistic and objective empathy with oneself and other women: The client increasingly develops a working knowledge of the personal and the divine so that she can take responsibility for what is truly personal, and realistically disavow responsibility for her fate, that which seems to happen because of luck, opportunity, or accident. This goal, an extension of work at earlier stages, should result in a sense of objectivity in the client's attitude toward herself in the moment and over time. This perspective should include sufficient understanding of broad interpersonal themes and values, and the ability to accept differences, especially in other women, with equanimity, or at least with tolerance.

6. An ability to appreciate how meanings, especially interpersonal meanings such as identity attributes for gender, intersect with broad political and social movements over time: Again, as an extension of the goals mentioned at earlier stages, a client now recognizes that meaning, both in attitudes and in values, is constructed out of social, interpersonal, biological, and psychological contexts. She begins to distinguish clearly between those concerns whose outcomes she can directly influence, such as her work and her expression of feeling life, and those

which she cannot control, such as her children's development or her husband's career. For women, this usually involves coming to terms with the political functions served by ideals of motherhood. Anxiety or other symptomatic tendencies to internalize these ideals can be understood as the product of social influence rather than of individual deviance. As Dally (1982) says, "Anxious mothers are the plague of all who work with them and their children. Anxiety in mothers seems to be one of the characteristics of our age. Yet it is abnormal for a mother not to be anxious. This paradox results from the falsity inherent in the idealization of motherhood that is so prevalent in Western society today. Our society pushes the concept of 'natural,' anxiety free motherhood while at the same time creating anxious mothers" (p. 249). Recognizing the paradoxical nature of mothering and motherhood can contribute to developing a lively humor and a taste for the absurd, as a broad appreciation for symbols.

All in all, these goals can be collapsed into the idea that therapist and client engender an analytic attitude and a perspective that allows the client to continue integrating unconscious and conflicting meaning for the rest of her life. When she feels free to do this with her own authentic voice and authority, she has then established a partnership with her animus. Similarly, she will be free to develop relationships of mutuality and equality with men in her life context. She will no longer try to constrain the personal attitudes, beliefs, or creations of men into the shape of her projected animus.

As we mentioned before, near the beginning of therapy with clients at this stage, we have frequently encountered dreams that include a fantastic or divine child. Archetypally we interpret this kind of image as a signal of individuation, of the development of a uniquely creative personality in a life context of greater authority. Depending on the woman and the stresses which she is currently suffering, the divine child image may signal distant developmental potentials or immediate transformations. For clients at this stage, it is generally the latter. The following dream is from Diane who was described in Chapter 7.

Dream that I am having another baby. My husband is very lukewarm about it, but I am very excited. The hospital calls to say the baby has arrived and I am thrilled. We jump in the car and drive over. My husband has trouble with the directions, but I *know* the way. There is a backup line of parents waiting to see babies. It is all very businesslike; babies are cataloged, nurses are brisk. I can see the boxes full of babies all in a line and can spot mine well in advance. I tell my husband that I feel like a mother cat being able to spot her own litter, because this tiny, tiny—about eight inches long—baby looks exactly like all the others did, only more alert. She will be very pretty and seems to recognize us. Round head, lots of hair, small perfect features. I am absolutely thrilled and open my jacket to nurse her. The nurse stands by watching as I adjust my huge nipple to her tiny, tiny mouth. She is so small that it is going to be hard—but I am an experienced mother. Very patient. She finally takes some of the first fluids and gets interested. This is a long process. Will she engage to the nipple? Will she nurse? She does! I can take her home!

In the dream, the name of the baby is given to the dreamer over the telephone when the hospital calls. The name connects the infant to an earlier dream figure, a Black man who is a Dionysian figure for the dreamer. This baby seems to have been fathered by him and it is through nursing her that the dreamer gets sexually excited. (Sexual apathy was a presenting problem.) The dream continues:

While waiting for the nurse to wrap her up for me, I notice that I am sexually excited. I am ready for action now that the baby has come; I can be sexually active again.

In the therapeutic session, Diane and her therapist reflected on the style of the therapeutic relationship, which was depicted in the dream. Diane had experienced the therapist as "extremely businesslike" and "very busy." These qualities come across in the routines of the hospital and the manner of the nurse. Diane had been hoping that her therapist would be "more nurturant and supportive" and that she (Diane) might finally experience herself as "being mothered" by an authority, a female authority. Helping Diane contain her desire to be literally mothered, the therapist laughed with her about the degree of "objectivity" depicted in the hospital and nursing staff, suggesting to Diane that she might assume greater objectivity in her own attitude about her development.

Her new baby is perfect, though very tiny, and Diane can clearly nurture it herself. Diane perceived this idea as a positive turn because she had so long assumed that she "had no thinking function" and that the strength of rationality or objectivity had to come from her husband. Over the years, she had complained that he "lacked strength" and that she could not lean on him for any kind of foundation or support. Instead of Diane embracing the Bear Man (the earlier heroic animus) or the Dionysian Black man in herself, she had always attempted to find him in her husband. Through increasing her belief in her own ability to think objectively, Diane eventually withdrew this projection from her husband and wrote a publishable paper from her own perspective. Her husband was actually quite a reliable, accomplished man, but his personal style of relating was simply different from Diane's heroic animus.

Motherhood and marriage are often the symbolic arenas in which women confront their distortions, wishes, and hopes for individuation, even these later stages. Being the daughter of a mother continues to be a central identity theme for personal transformation over adult phases and stages of development. The condition of being female in a patriarchal society always includes contractual and political arrangements with the fathers of the culture. These arrangements tend to be organized around these two institutions in which women are contractually bonded to men to perform a variety of duties under the supervision, and willful influence and even possession, of men. In a different society, the image of individuation might be different, but in ours, women must come to terms with the boundaries and constraints of their contracts with the patriarchy as they attempt to restore female authority to consciousness.

The following dream exhibits the complexity and extraordinary quality of symbolic imagery that typify the dreams of women in the later animus stages. Many levels of meaning compete as opposites intersect in this depiction of a sacred marriage. The dream is from Alma, a woman in her mid-30s, who entered therapy at the Autonomous Stage of ego development. She had been a creative and industrious career woman throughout most of her adult life, but she had not formed trusting relationships with men. Her presenting problem in therapy, an inability to trust men, was often manifested in aggressive responses to males at times when Alma desired their protection and support. The dream:

A young boy and girl are betrothed. The boy is very much in love with the girl, but the girl seems a little indifferent. Perhaps it is what she must go through to get married.

The marriage ceremony with the priest is centered around a huge stone altar. The virgin must be strapped to the altar in front of the priest and the girl's family, and the marriage must be consummated in front of them. After consummation, the priest and the mother go upstairs to have sex while the father takes care of the children. Soon the father follows the mother to see what is going on.

The boy wants to have sex again. When he thinks of the mother and the priest, he spontaneously has an orgasm; he has sperm all over. The girl wipes it off. The scene changes and the girl is naked on a different altar in another room. The boy seems to have turned mean. He is standing over her and says he is going to give her an abortion. "This is a bitch day!!" he says. There are all sorts of boiling, steaming medieval instruments in a laboratory. He will give the girl an abortion as punishment.

As an observer in the dream, I don't understand because this seems to be incongruent with his previous commitment to love her. I close my eyes. I cannot watch. When I open my eyes, the fetus is lying on the altar. It is very much in one piece, covered with afterbirth. I am amazed how large it is. It just looks like a perfect baby, not a fetus at all. Then something miraculous happens. The baby gets up and walks around the altar. It even speaks, saying something like "I can't believe this is happening." It has a man's head but an infant body. Then it looks up and there is a blue stained-glass window over its head, radiating white light on the infant. The infant has a white glow around it.

The infant then crawls down from the large altar to a small pedestal with a statue of the Virgin Mother on it. The statue radiates the light also and it is outlined in a glow. The infant now grows into a small boy. I reach out and pull an even larger statue of the Virgin from behind the altar. It too is glowing with white light.

The Virgin Mother is an androgynous symbol of a female who can generate her own development independently of a male. She has realized both masculine and feminine potentials and has combined strength and compassion in her unique form of power. Prior to the Middle Ages, the meaning of *virgin* did not include the idea of chastity. Rather, the virgin (as with the vestal virgin) was a woman who belonged to no single male partner. She was free and independent of masculine possession.

The dream presents a confusing array of rather violent and promising images which the therapist and client sorted through. Alma had sustained abuse at the hands of men in waking life, and it was fitting that her divine child should be delivered through an abortion. Her own sexual development had, indeed, been aborted. This had been her fate. The meaning that Alma could take from this—that the abuse had not simply been a loss but was now an avenue to deeper connections with herself—was a promising avenue of development. Similarly, her abuse connected her empathically with the suffering of other women and with a desire to change a society that so abuses its members. The threat of male aggression (the abortion) becomes the transforming influence as the girl submits to the ordeal. Thus, Alma actively submitted to a deeper understanding of her own repressions, as difficult as they were to face directly. Alma's transformation took place more internally than externally. She learned to trust her own animus complex and to believe in the process of her development, even though it was grounded in a tragic event. On the other hand, Alma did not come to trust men in her interpersonal life, in that she recognized how little control she had over a man's true commitment to a caring relationship with her.

Trusting men is, of course, a focal theme at this fourth stage. When a woman has recognized her inherent worthiness (she becomes a *goddess* from the image in the theme story), she questions how much she can interact with men in her environment, who may continue to project patriarchal female themes (*anima complex*, in Jungian terminology) onto her actions and desires. Some women may conclude just at the point at which they are truly ready for mutual partnership that men they know are not to be trusted because they are not evolved developmentally. We work with women to withdraw the projected animus—whether it is a rapist, a god, a critic, a hero, or a father—but we cannot guarantee that our clients will find suitable partners either in the men they have married or among the men they know. When women discriminate their own masculine potentials, they no longer expect men to be versions of animus ideals. Instead they accept great differences between men and women as an aspect of our contemporary condition. That a woman may not find men who have similar insight can seem like a great loss at this point because, of course, she is not relieved of her need and desire for male companionship. She may be more comfortable with *both men and women*, but she still desires intimacy—with a man if she is heterosexual or with a woman if she is lesbian—and will have to grieve its loss if she cannot find a loving partner.

Ironically, then, the theme of abandonment sometimes becomes real and concrete as women transform themselves and discover their best potentials. Still, the strength and courage of a woman's integration will continue to grow in the face of such a loss. Therapists should be informed, however, that a side effect of a woman's further development can sometimes to be the loss of an intimate partner who refuses to go on developing.

The integration of the animus complex in analytic therapy is ultimately the securing of a symbolic life. As a woman continues an internal dialogue with her own complexes, she will expand her personal identity and enlarge her sense of authority. Anxieties about competing roles and attitudes will not seem overwhelming. Integrating her own maleness permits her greater prominence and courage in a patriarchal culture. Integrating her own aggression releases energy to express and defend her needs.

Still, some women who have achieved the integration of animus feel ambivalent about their achievement. This ambivalence must be acknowledged as reasonable in a patriarchal society. Fostering development in oneself—or in another—is not always rewarding. Resistance to change, fear of repeating traumas, reluctance to be an outsider, and guilt about hurting others are necessarily a part of individuation, which forces us repeatedly to accept the limitations of our humanity.

ANIMUS AS ANDROGYNE

With the idea that any developmental scheme is "open" or potentially inadequate, we have included a final stage, which is sketched in terms of ideals for female development. Certainly we do not know what the future holds or what kind of personality may be slowly evolving through the evolution of human consciousness. We do, however, have some ideas about the "truly integrated" personality for women. A few seem to achieve a freedom from fears of betrayal, abandonment, and imperfection. They seem wholly to trust in the process of their own growth and in the constantly emerging fabrics of relationships in their lives. In our terms, we would say they have achieved an *objective empathy.*

Empathy, the power to intuit reality accurately and then to "move with" another's reality, is a concept fundamental to our entire developmental scheme. The following dream is from Andrea, whose material was reported in Chapter 7. Andrea was 35 when she had the dream. She had been in analytic therapy for almost 5 years at that time. Although Andrea had not yet achieved a final integration of animus, the dream depicted a potential that was startling to both client and therapist. This dream continued to be a landmark experience for Andrea as she changed in the ensuing years. The dream depicts the power of empathy as an "organic will" that influences the physical world at the level of submolecular structures. This is a will which moves things without pushing them.

I am working in the Women's Self Help Center, where I am actively involved in projects that have a positive aim for all women. I feel that my energy is essential to the well-being of the organization.

Someone brings me an old scraggly pine branch and presents it as a precious gift. I am puzzled by this solemn affair, but concentrate on the branch and find that I can move it psychokinetically without touching it. If I concentrate on moving the branch, it sways gently as if a breeze were blowing. I recognize that my *gift* is making things move without mechanically pushing them. I notice that I can move any object in this way if I choose to concentrate.

I think to myself that this gift has no real purpose. What could be gained by arbitrarily moving things about through one's psychic powers? Besides, I can immediately see the possibility for the corruption of this kind of power.

I consult with a physicist about the phenomenon of psychokinesis. He comes to witness my ability. He tells me very solemnly that this is a great gift which has a name. It is called the *organic will.* This is a will that stems from consciousness at a submolecular level, resulting in a subtle rearrangement of protons, neutrons, and electrons into new molecular structures toward a transformation of matter. Hence, what appears to be movement at the level of the phenomenal world is transformation of matter itself through the organic will. I am deeply impressed and wake up.

A few remarks on this dream will expand its meaning. The pine branch is a symbol for Dionysus, something known by the dreamer. Dionysus, as the androgynous male god and the partner of Ariadne, appears as a "moving force" in the dreamer's gift. The strength of the dreamer's consciousness is depicted as firmly rooted in the subleties of the natural world. Her gift of *organic will* indicates the ability to move the world through her own responsible consciousness. The type of consciousness, deeply bound to the structure of the physical or perceived world, can be interpreted as an example of *objective empathy*. Such an empathy is experienced subjectively as expanded awareness and control. The person feels more adequate and more alive than at earlier stages.

Futhermore, the dream depicts a kind of objectivity or accuracy of inference that goes beyond rational explanation. This kind of objectivity, intuitively reflecting on the nature of things "as they are," may be an extension of human awareness made possible through very attentive, enduring relationships with the human and natural worlds, relationships of the sort women especially learn to engender.

ANIMUS DEVELOPMENT: THE SCHEME

What we have presented in our discussions of the stages of animus development (Chaps. 5–8) is a heuristic for a model of assessment and treatment of women in psychotherapy. Our focus is empowerment, the development of authority and empathy in a patriarchal society.

Combining social and symbolic psychologies to move toward a new psychology of female development seems to us to be a promising orientation. A Jungian developmental approach to symbolic interpretation lends a new perspective to data gathered from social psychological studies. Interpreting from a mythological, literary, or artistic perspective, as Jung does, allows one to focus on the universal, the archaic, the common sense, and the enduring in human life. Sometimes we can anticipate a "future solution" by using a map of universal themes in human consciousness. On the other hand, we are aware that we have to be careful to put into context our understanding of myths and stories, of artistic images and religious rites. We cannot assume that the myth of Pandora, for example, conveys to us a "universal" theme that we are not actively constructing.

More reductive forms of interpretation—working from the client's own associations to her past—help us understand the context of the client's immediate culture (interpersonal world), and they balance the archetypal point of view. Often clients focus automatically on what was "wrong" or "missing" in early environments. A life story is constructed which sounds like a series of disappointments, abandonments, rejections—or else the story sounds ideal, but the person's own actions are disappointing, problematic, wrong, etc.

Rather than focusing on what is defective, archetypal interpretation focuses on meaning and purpose. "What is the purpose of this dream or image right now? Why this one instead of some other?" A hopeful orientation toward expanding symbolic meaning encourages a dialectical stance regarding inner processes. Making use of both rational and nonrational thought forms, in penetrating the troubles of life, results in expanded imagination and a more hopeful attitude leading to better problem solving.

Looking back over the stories we have presented to illuminate the female personality, we see certain threads of meaning that provide connections among the stories. A major theme is regaining trust in female "intuition." Persephone's reaching out for the narcissus flower was an intuitive grasping at the natural world of beauty. Pandora's curiosity about the inside of the earthenware jar was a premature or impulsive turn to inner suffering. Psyche's lighting of the candle over Amor's body was a jealous investigation of a powerful male reality. Ariadne's conscious journey into the labyrinth was a courageous confrontation with the aggressive and powerful monster who was her own brother, the product of her mother's angry copulation.

Ariadne offers a special lesson in terms of modern feminism. She recognized the necessity, as it were, of saving the children and the race of humans by annihilating the corrupt form of feminism represented in the minotaur. The white bull, father of the minotaur, was the creature sent to Crete by Poseidon. This creature can be interpreted as mythologically connected with the great Bull of Heaven which Gilgamesh slew in the Babylonian epic. The bull represents the power of the earlier matriarchal culture of fertility. The bull went "underground" during the long period of patriarchal domination of culture. Female power was maligned, buried, hidden, and considered evil. The natural procreative powers of women were uncelebrated and denigrated. Reconnection to the Bull of Heaven, and hence the rightful powers of women, was too hastily or prematurely enacted by Pasiphae when she mated with the white bull. Such a reconnection, Ariadne would suggest, must be accomplished through consciousness rather than through impulse.

Ariadne was punished for the death of her brother by being dumped on an obscure island by a national hero. Like Gilgamesh after the death of the Bull of Heaven, Ariadne's energy is expended on her heroic deed and she is left to die. But unlike Gilgamesh, she has performed a compassionate deed, not an individual heroic task, and therefore she is transformed, awakened by her own androgynous god, and is completed in her nature as a divinity.

For modern women, there is no wholly adequate story for the integration of animus. The old matriarchal myths have been largely buried and lost to us. The Greek and Roman stories take us only partway—perhaps because the edge of our consciousness is still unfolding. Through poets and dreamers, however, we catch a glimpse of the steady gaze of the integrated woman who has a serene confidence in her own abilities. The concluding lines of Adrienne Rich's (1984a) poem "Diving into the Wreck" seem to us to depict such a state of mind:

> We are, I am, you are
> by cowardice or courage
> the ones who find our way
> back to this scene
> carrying a knife, a camera
> a book of myths
> in which our names do not appear.
> (Rich, 1984a)

9

Pandora: Identity Relationship in Adulthood

Offering the story of an actual person who is going through psychotherapy presents many risks, both for the client and for the reader. Any
time we seek to make a case study out of an individual life, we naturally
obscure some of what is essential about a person's individuality in order
to protect her identity. The risk for the client is that what she reads may
be harmful, or at least not helpful in terms of her insight and satisfaction. The risk for the reader is knowing both too much and too little, so that disentangling the general categories for conceptualizing a
case from the particulars of a life history may be difficult, if not impossible. Still, psychotherapists have traditionally learned new methods and
discovered new ideas through sharing case material, much in the for-
mat presented here.

The person who is herein called "Pandora" has graciously given
her consent to our presentation of the material of this chapter. She
realizes that "Pandora" is certainly not a complete description of her,
nor of the process of therapy with her, but rather that it is a story told
with the intention of exposing a particular perspective on her psychotherapy, the therapist's conception of it. The case was handled by
Young-Eisendrath.

Pandora's case is presented with a desire for the kind of understanding that is accurate and helpful for others as the basis for dialogue.
Consequently, I have presented it in two chapters, the first of which
emphasizes assessment and personality functioning throughout much
of the therapeutic process. This first chapter was written as part of an
ongoing therapy with Pandora, before she moved away to another city. Specifically, I wanted to illustrate the way in which I use the concepts we have set forth in the chapter on the Pandora Stage of animus
functioning.

The second chapter presents some direct evidence from my encounter with Pandora. It is primarily a transcript of the 110th session in her psychotherapy. This transcript includes all interchanges verbatim (except those features that might expose Pandora's actual identity; there were only a few). Alongside the verbatim transcript are my comments on what I assume was taking place between us during this session. Since Pandora has read all of this material and offered her corrections and insights, I can say that she finds my report "congruent enough" with her experiences not to be troubled. Also in the second chapter is the conclusion of the case and a brief "epilogue" about what took place in the final months of her treatment, after the manuscript for this book had been completed and Pandora had read about her own case. The rationale for including this second chapter is an educational one. If therapists are to have a dialogue of shared meaning, we need to see more complete accounts of each others' work than the usual case summaries which are primarily shaped around the therapist's conceptual biases.

In terms of the language and images of animus development, I have been striving to help this woman become more of an "equal partner" with men in projects she desires to do—more of a Psyche whose own curiosity will lead her out of anxious depression and a diminishing sense of self-worth. She and I have not yet arrived at the point at which Pandora's enthusiastic curiosity can lead her forward. Rather, we have been absorbed in the confrontation with the "buried feminine" in the earthenware jar. My client fears that she does not have the strength to really look within. Alternately, she is afraid that the jar is empty. Our struggles together are especially, and sometimes beautifully, illustrative of the ordinary struggles of younger women to believe in themselves, in their own intelligence, and in their ability to run their own lives. Because of the demands this struggle makes on my imagination, I have chosen this case to illustrate both the strengths and weaknesses of my work as a psychotherapist.

To obscure the personal identity of my client while remaining true to the essential material of the case, I will change the details of her life situation as I expose some of the aspects of our work. Both her dreams and a full-length dialogue from a therapy session are presented largely intact as they occurred. The actual identifying factors of this woman's personality are also intact, while the facts of her age, occupation, and appearance are changed. These details are presented in a way that is "close enough," I believe, to the facts of the case to avoid misrepresenting our work together.

Pandora was 28 years old when she entered therapy with me. She has been with me for almost 2½ years, meeting once a week. In my notes from my initial session, I have said that her "presenting problem" was depression over the recent loss of her boyfriend, whom I will call "Dan." Because Pandora knew a great deal about the language of psychotherapy, she mentioned "fears of abandonment" connected not only to losing Dan, but also to her parents' plans to move out of the United States after her father's retirement. Pandora had recently moved from New England to Philadelphia in order to take a new administrative position of some responsibility. The move had been precipitated by her decision not to finish her dissertation for a PhD in Education, although finishing it would have given her the freedom to change careers, to become a psychotherapist, which had been her long-term goal.

Because her family of origin lived in a nearby state, she saw herself as "coming back" to the environment of her childhood. She believed that her new employment, which provided a substantial salary, was a move toward "financial independence" and "self-reliance." As a graduate student, she had felt too "dependent" on others' approval and authority. Actually, she had achieved a great deal in graduate school and had been awarded scholarships for her work, had been encouraged by her mentors, and had been perceived as a leader by other students.

In the initial session, Pandora looked back over her life's story with some despair about her future. She saw herself as "avoiding making real decisions" in the past and as drifting from opportunity to opportunity without any sense of what she really wanted. She described herself as the product of other peoples' influence and she was visibly distressed about this. Her earlier employment and her college major just seemed to "happen to her." We came up with an image that she humorously embraced to characterize herself: She had been "a hitchhiker at the side of life."

Pandora was self-disparaging about her accomplishments. She believed that others saw potentials in her that were not real. Secretly, she felt that she "wasn't very bright" and that her apparent ability for leadership was bravado. She was tired of "fooling other people" into believing that she could really do something with her life.

Most aggravating to her sense of herself had been the recent breakup with Dan. She had met him in graduate school, where, initially, he had pursued her. He thought she was a strong woman, stronger than he, and he had an idealized image of what she could bring him. "He wanted a mother and someone who would bolster him and tell him how good and smart and strong he could be. It was depressing, really, at first, and I just couldn't see much in him." After several months of his pursuit, however, she "gave in" and decided to "see what was there" in a committed relationship to him. Gradually she and Dan became a couple who were recognized socially and invited out together.

Finally she "gave over completely" to the relationship and began to imagine some future life together. Life as a couple was not easy, however. She felt that Dan "just could not give." She said he was willing to talk endlessly about himself and his own problems, but he was reluctant to help Pandora.

Her move to Philadelphia was in part a reaction to the relationship. She wanted "more space" and financial freedom so that she could decide how she would map her future. If she married Dan, she wanted the marriage to be her own decision, and if she did not marry him, she wanted to be securely on her own. A part of her plan was to have an "active weekend relationship" with Dan, who could come down to the City and "play" with her on a regular basis. After she moved, he visited several times. Then she took him to a family gathering, on an important family holiday, and presented him as her "beau." She was very proud of this, being the youngest of four children and the last to secure a boyfriend. Immediately after the family gathering, on the same night in fact, he told her he wanted to break off their relationship. He wanted freedom to get involved with other women, and he did not see much future in traipsing back and forth between graduate school and Philadelphia. She felt abandoned, enraged, and punished.

Preoccupied with thoughts that she had sabotaged the "only good relationship she had ever had," she obsessively examined her motivations to move away from New England. For 3 months before she contacted me, she thought about "getting back into therapy." (She had previously been in therapy with another psychologist and had found it "very helpful.") Although she knew about me through a friend and had decided to call me several times, she did not "want to become dependent on therapy for figuring out" what she wanted in her life. Finally, however, she could no longer tolerate the anxiety of her obsessive self-examination.

One more strand of her story deserves mention, as part of the presenting problem. She had quickly come to view her new job as "a drag." Administrative work seemed empty compared to graduate school, and she felt a developing hostility between her boss, "Bill," and herself. She believed that Bill did not see her strengths as a planner or a salesperson and that he was competitive with her abilities. She felt that her job was "not using her talents," and she wanted out although she had barely begun.

The only satisfaction she felt from her return to her environment of childhood was the reunion with her family of origin. She respected her brother and sisters and loved being around her parents. Family gatherings had become the core of social life and she was "desperately afraid" of what would happen after her parents moved out of the country.

ASSESSMENT

Pandora's strengths were many, although they were not claimed in her self-concept. She had been earning her own way in the world since the age of 18 and had held many responsible positions. She was articulate, witty, and urbane in her self-presentation, and I found myself "enjoying" our first sessions together. Her energy level and physical activities did not display a "depressed" pattern, nor did she appear to be "manic" or overly occupied with "doing." I admired her ability to enjoy pleasure in her leisure time. She was recognized as a "life of the party," by both her family and her friends. She had established a support network of women and men, both at her new job and at graduate school.

In conversation she was quite knowledgeable about her fields of study, but she saw herself as a beginner potentially unsuited to her career goals. She said she was "afraid" of the real tests of her profession although she wanted to practice psychotherapy and to attain a respectable status.

In terms of her appearance, she also seemed competent. She presented herself in a stylish, collegiate, and casual kind of dress, which fitted well with her age and personality. She was at an attractive weight, and she looked physically fit (although she wanted to lose weight initially). Her gestures and facial expressions were congruent with her emotions, and she made effective use of body movements in expressing herself.

Pandora's vulnerabilities could be seen more clearly in her personal family history than in her self-presentation. As the youngest of four children, she had always feared being ignored or abandoned by those in authority. Furthermore, she had grown up in a traditional Catholic family with a strong ethnic orientation. When she separated from her family to join her peers, she felt bereft of the clear and concrete guidelines that tradition had provided. Throughout her childhood, she had constantly identified with the strengths and success of her older sister (about a year and a half older), "Emma." When Pandora left home, she also left behind the guiding reflection of Emma, whom she had incessantly "copied" during childhood, in dress and manner.

More important than her departure from the clear guidelines of tradition and the example her older sister provided, however, were her parental complexes. Mother was "weak, depressed, bitter" and emotionally unavailable. Pandora described long periods of time when her mother would not speak to members of the family. Apparently, her mother would say "I'm going into my shell" and withdraw into an obvious depression. Mother did not openly express anger, but seemed to "burn slowly" with resentment and bitterness. At the time she entered therapy, Pandora's active Mother complex, as she had internalized it, was a "shell." Nothing strong, good, or definite was attached to this complex, and Pandora struggled constantly to differentiate herself from it.

Whereas the Mother complex was weak and shallow, the Father was strong and aggressive. Father was described as domineering, intelligent, articulate, argumentative, and a tease. He was witty, but competitive with his children, constantly "tricking" them with some riddle or puzzle and then glowing with triumph over his defeat of their intelligence. Father sought achievement and power, financial success, and cultural sophistication, but he fell short at all of them. By Pandora's description, he had managed a fairly successful independent business and was a self-made man of immigrant parents, but he had not achieved all that he had hoped for. His special desire was recognition of his intelligence and his quick wit.

Vulnerability to being overwhelmed by and identifying with this domineering Father was the major issue that I anticipated in our work. Naturally, her vulnerability to being shaped and defeated by the Father would emerge most prominently in intimate relationships with men, and in subordinate relationships with male authority figures.

Stresses in my client's current life situation exacerbated these vulnerabilities considerably and interfered with her competences. The uprooting caused by a major move to another city and a new job would have precipitated abandonment fears in any young woman, and added to these stresses was the return to her family of origin prior to her securing adult status. Once back with her actual father, Pandora became vulnerable to feeling overwhelmed by what she perceived as his speical requests for intimacies with her. She believed that she was a "special confidante" of Father, who could not adequately work through his feeling life without her. When she would approach her own father with this orientation, however, she would typically find that he disappointed her by caring little about her life, and only complaining about his.

From the intrapsychic point of view, I anticipated that our work would center around discriminating Pandora's real strengths and interests. Furthermore, I knew we would have to analyze the Father complex as we were strengthening the Mother.

From the interpersonal point of view, I could anticipate my client's suspicion and her resistance to me. I would not be a good-enough Mother initially because she had so many genuine doubts about the strength and competence of women. Either she would imagine that I was really a "Father type" who was manipulating my way around the world and was therefore unavailable to understand her, or that some man was backing me up and providing for me so that I could look good in the world. I did not know what form her resistance would take, but I could anticipate a strong ambivalence.

From the point of view of her ego development, I assessed Pandora to be in the throes of the Self-Aware Stage. Pandora's conscious desires to be logical and rational, and to formulate her own goals were preoccupations that signal the Self-Aware Stage. Talking about personal goals and personal feelings is rewarding in itself at this stage, and Pandora loved to talk about them. Quoting from Chapter 4:

> Because she has no coherently established self-concept, and because she has externalized authority and internalized inferiority, the woman feels acute pressure about her desire to find herself. Although she may not verbally state her anxiety about old standards of appearance and values, she will appear pressured when making decisions about changing her life-style, her orientation, and her appearance. (p. 60)

Vulnerable to depression and acute anxiety, a woman at this stage can experience profound lack of control because of the unpredictability of anxiety over low self-esteem. Giving over her identity to the animus complex can result in excessive pressure to find a direction. She is vulnerable to enacting goals and motivations which are not her own (Father complex) and to feeling badgered by internal (especially male) voices which critically judge everything she does. The inner conflicts between female identity and animus complex emerge initially at the Self-Aware Stage in a woman's conscious awareness (earlier, they are predominately acted out).

From ego development research, we know that women at this stage are also inclined to retreat into earlier modes of self-protection and into defensive reactions that are ineffective for further development. The defenses typical of the Self-Aware Stage include projection of feelings, rationalization, reaction formation, and repression. These rather "high-level" defenses can be regressively replaced by projective identification, some milder forms of splitting, and denial.

Finally, from the point of view of psychopathology, I would assess Pandora as having an identity disorder of adolescence in adulthood. Although some features of borderline personality emerge in an intense identity disorder, they neither predominate nor disrupt interpersonal relationships as they would in the case of a true borderline disorder. Pandora shows evidence of high-level ego functioning in several areas of her life and presents an identity that is typical for many young women in our culture.

GOALS OF THERAPY

Our initial goals were to help Pandora clarify her career decisions, in the context of understanding her identification with Father. We decided to work on separating her own desires from the wishes and fears she carried from childhood.

I recommended that we work both analytically and behaviorally, which I prefer to do when I am working to achieve some independence from overwhelming animus and parental complexes. On the analytical side, we would interpret dreams and therapeutic relationship in the light of symbolic meaning, especially regarding her self-esteem and motivation. On the behavioral side, we would formulate "agreements" or "assignments" for actual behavioral change outside of therapy and monitor these in some kind of empirical way. For example, we used the behavioral technique of *thought stopping* and she kept track of her responses.

Separation and differentiation from the powerful Father complex was the general developmental goal of her therapy.

PROCESS OF THERAPY

Pandora, of course, had always longed for a mother and comforter, someone strong enough to just let Pandora "be." If I were to enact this kind of symbiotic mothering at this point in her development, however, we would tend to drown in a sea of possibilities or "just be in her feelings." So we began our work on separation (and individuation) with the ambivalent longing for Mother. Our goals focused us on the future and career. Her initial dream in therapy expresses both her desires to become a psychotherapist and her ambivalence about it:

A male friend (H) and I went to a Jungian seminar. It was filled mostly with therapists that were getting advanced training. A young woman, dressed in a blouse and a skirt, walked up a flight of stairs into this rather dimly lit old room. After the seminar H and I decided to kiss outside and we touched mouths, but didn't "french kiss." He was thrilled that we could kiss, and he was turned on. I was surprised that he was turned on because he was never attracted to me for a sexual relationship. I thought it was strange to just kiss and not further it. He was excited that this could open up a whole new dimension to the relationship.

Although she quickly "enters" the Jungian framework, the room is unimpressive, and she escapes to more exciting sexual contact. She "decided to kiss outside," and initially she kept me running after her, as she had kept her lovers running until they caught her.

In many Pandora women, I have found that the initial problem in therapy centers around either getting a man or becoming a man. Because they do not trust me initially to be a good-enough Mother, they focus on my capacity to father them. Part of the wished-for fathering seems to be that I will deliver them into the arms of a man, as the father does in the wedding ceremony. If ongoing relationships with men are not working out or a promising new one is not on the horizon, we have problems of trust before we can cooperate in a therapeutic alliance.

With Pandora, these showed up in the third session when she announced to me that she was going back to New England. She contended that only in New England would she be happy and that perhaps she could finish her doctorate and marry Dan. When I examined the reality of this proposal, however, there was little in it. Dan had a girlfriend and Pandora had no idea for a topic for her dissertation. I told her that I thought her plans were based on fear and fantasy, and that I could not support the move, although she was obviously free to go.

For about a month, she attempted to move. She made a connection for a job interview in New England. During this time her therapy was on hold and she would say "I don't know for sure if I will be here next week or not." Finally the job possibility fell through, and she was faced with me in her future. In confronting her situation she had the following dream:

Skating on what was supposedly thin ice that turned out to be thin ice. People fell in and I am not sure if I did or not, but I was trying to help people out of the water. It was a *crisis*.

I interpreted the dream in a positive fashion, emphasizing both her subjective experience of saving people who were drowning inside and her capacity to become a psychotherapist, her career goal.

She decided to stay in therapy and work through the separation from her parents. The next day she had the following dream:

I was held hostage with others in a small, cramped house. The man who was watching me was going to lose his mind and I was able to help him by seducing him, forcing myself on him. Both of us were sweating and in a very cramped area. He managed his "break" and didn't go crazy. It was culminated by sex, but the intensity of my pressure seemed more significant than the sex. After this climax, we were very relieved and I was relieved to have been able to help. (The man was dark, like my father, and looked like someone I know. I woke up feeling disturbed for dreaming what seemed to be "regressive.")

I realized that she might feel I was pressuring her to "grow up" too fast. She continued to seek comfort in a Pandora identity, to find a male to validate her worth. She also continued to have problems with "Bill" (her boss) although they took a different turn.

At work, she began to campaign for change in the environment by articulating her own values. I was supportive and did considerable behavioral contracting with her about realistic strategies for realizing her ideals. In the end, she gained some positive attention for these, but the environment was such that her desires could not be wholly actualized. She had to accept something less than a compromise. Still, the involvement in a cooperative "project" together seemed to bind her to me in a different way, and I began to feel a therapeutic alliance evolving around the central concerns of her own development. At about this time, she had the following dream (eighth session in therapy):

Went to a male doctor and he detected a lump on my left breast. He wanted to operate immediately, and I was horrified by his assumption that I would willingly just have this operation. I found him rough and pompous, and I told him that I was seeking a female doctor. He had a very condescending attitude and said, "Sure, go ahead, but she'll not be as good as I am." He was very indignant that I had questioned his authority.

She associated the rough intrusiveness of this male doctor with her own father. He had often attempted to help her by intruding on her individuality or freedom. We began to analyze her Father complex, trying to understand how and when it incapacitated her in her daily activities. The lump on her left breast was interpreted as the fear of some hidden disease or flaw in her femininity, and the male doctor's response seemed to be that this flaw should be excised by him, in his way. In fact, she had had many hormonal difficulties and had encountered some male doctors of this type. Her fantasized flaw took the form of believing that she was too weak and too empty to support any kind of relationship, either to herself or to a man. From the point of view of her conscious identity, she was a strong, independent woman among her friends, but she feared that she was only playing a role.

During the first 8 months of our work, Pandora made many changes in her life context. She claimed her apartment as her home and decorated it in her own way. She moved her piano out of her parents' home and into her apartment (she was an accomplished pianist), and she began to feel settled in her new life.

Repeatedly she decided to do something about her dissertation, but then would not follow through. She contacted her adviser and discovered that the adviser was departing the university, and thus she would be reassigned. In each session we struggled anew with problems of motivation, Pandora feeling bored with her corporate work and yet not ready to follow her own desire.

Throughout the first year in therapy, Pandora slowly gained confidence that she could survive quite well on her own after her parents' move. She came to feel more secure in local friendships and better about her job (although never satisfied, especially with Bill). She began to see feminism as a valued orientation in her personal life. While all of these themes were slowly unfolding, I would feel impatient about her career development, and she would be anxious about not finding a man. Many of her dreams would compensate the absence of a male partner by providing her the opportunity for contact with an attractive man. The following dream was typical:

I met the man who wanted to have a relationship with me at an office-type party. He was very nervous to be seen with me at the party, yet he stayed near and told me how he truly wanted to be with me. He was married and he tried to call his wife from the restaurant where the party was held, but didn't reach her. I was very attracted to him and felt very excited by the intrigue. I wanted to know his whole life, about his relationships. He was a nice-looking, preppy-dressed man. I was nicely dressed too and looked very well.

I had the clear impression that I was pulling this woman in one direction while her animus complex was pulling in another. No matter how often we reviewed the circumstances of her early fathering, of her mother's depression and despair, of her father's competition for attention, and her irrational messages to herself about being fat and stupid, Pandora did not move toward her own creative work. She did contact male friends and sometimes had a weekend of sex and partying. These contacts tended to have the character of college dating, and no strong alliance emerged. At the same time, she would turn to me fairly often and say, "Should I contact Dan?" and recount a fantasized dialogue she had had with him or something she just "had to find out."

Finally I supported her desire to meet Dan in person, at a restaurant in a distant city. After an identity relationship has ended, a woman's own conscious identity must be strengthened and separated from the man onto whom she projected her animus before she can potentially benefit from returning "to the scene of the crime."

When she returned to visit Dan she discovered a man much weaker than the one she remembered. She called him "narcissistic" and found him to be wholly unconnected to her emotionally. Still she had difficulty withdrawing her projection because of his sensitive manner and good looks. The realistic withdrawal of her animus projection onto Dan actually occurred a few months into the second year of therapy. After her visit with Dan, Pandora began to shape her current life more enthusiastically. She was involved in her new friendships and giving thought to a practice in psychotherapy and even to returning to her dissertation. At work things were better, too. She was able to handle Bill more effectively and to accept some of his criticism. She was beginning to internalize some of her own competence, although the separation from her parents continued to frighten her. The following dream characterizes some of the changes in her conscious identity and a greater integration of her own responsibility and sexuality.

I was accompanying on the piano a musical play. A friend was accompanying the group also. The director yelled at me for playing so roughly, and I came to my own defense—that is, that it was the first time I had seen the music, but I also knew it was my responsibility. One fellow came over to me to take my defense also; that is, he understood my position.

Next, I was dancing in front of lots of mirrors in a studio/bathroom. I was moved to masturbate. Before I did, I woke up.

The self-stimulation expressed in the masturbation image is generally a positive sign of a woman's expression of sexuality and responsibility for satisfying her own sexual needs. In this case, the masturbation image was also connected to a fantasized specialness, of being the "chosen" daughter at the center of Father's attention, as we shall see.

Until this point in our therapy, I had not been aware of the wished-for specialness underlying this woman's pronounced sense of inferiority and denial of her own strengths. I had been encouraging her to work especially hard on appropriate respect for authority figures at work and on generating her own creative interests. Apparently, she felt that these "labors" should not be assigned to her. She wanted me to provode her access to supplies of status and creative interests in a protective, motherly way.

Only several months later did she express directly her anger at me for "not taking care of her feelings" and for "pushing too hard." Only recently did she reveal her anger that I had "brought my real daughter" (references to my daughter) into our therapy on several occasions in talking about Pandora. She also envied my relationship with my husband, assuming that my confidence and authority derived from my being grounded in his identity.

Pandora then met the man with whom she would have a consuming identity relationship. Her romantic involvement with him became the focus of our therapeutic work and has remained in center stage. She developed an identity relationship with "Bob," whose good looks and intelligence were compelling targets for the projection of her Hephaestian creative animus. Her fiercely possessive involvement with him is a prototype of an identity relationship.

An identity relationship is characterized by what appears to be a projection of a woman's entire self-concept onto a man. What previously might have been her own interests, appearance, or values now become bound to the man. The woman attempts to "remake" herself in the image which she believes he wants. In doing so, she anxiously watches his every look and gesture to see if he is appreciating her in proportion to her self-sacrifice. Obviously, he can never appreciate her to the degree that she wants because she has unconsciously given over her individuality to someone else's keeping. Eventually she will become enraged at his inattendance and attack him for the ways in which he repeats Father's offenses *and* the ways in which he does not emulate Father's strengths.

From a Jungian perspective, her identity is fused with the animus complex and then projected onto the man. The complex is inflated with all of her unlived idealism that belongs to excluded masculine power and creativity. The man who becomes the recipient of this projection is alternately inflated by the woman's expectations and deflated by her attacks on his actual performance.

Pandora's particular approach to the man of her dreams involved playing hard to get, in the sense that she offered a teasing and seemingly independent status of a "worldly woman" that her Father complex engendered. With Bob, she initially appeared to be a strong woman who would provide both intellectual stimulation and emotional play.

Bob is 8 years Pandora's junior. When they met, she appeared to be his superior in career and intellectual concerns. Indeed, she is more accomplished educationally and professionally, having pursued graduate work and earned a greater income. Bob was finishing undergraduate college and has only recently entered his profession. In the first month of their involvement, Pandora wondered whether he was too young and/or unsuited to her in terms of his ethnic and cultural background (which she sometimes viewed as inferior). Her early attraction was physical ("He is like a velvet horse in bed.") and power oriented ("He reminds me of one of those sweet punks from the movies, like John Travolta."). As she got to know him, she described him as "so sensitive" and "polite" and "old-fashioned" in the attention he gave her.

Almost immediately she recognized that her desires for Dan were now transferred to Bob. She worried about the intensity of these desires in the face of Bob's youthfulness, which might predispose him to polygamous needs. Here is a dream that occurred about a month after she met Bob. (She and Bob had begun having sex together after knowing each other a couple of weeks.)

I was sleeping in a double bed with Bob. Lying side by side, nestled. I picked my head up to see the dust on the headboard of the bed. I had a spray can in my hands, presumably a dust spray, and it started to spray uncontrollably. I couldn't control it. I handed him the can and he got the lid back on.

If we interpret the dust as unattended fall-out from other relatiohships on the "head" side of her situation, we can take the spray can to represent her emotional response both to the present relationship and to the worry about the past. Bob apparently could "put the lid on" her feelings better than she could. After about a month with him, she did indeed begin to feel out of control.

Pandora's meeting Bob occurred a few weeks prior to her parent's departure. Pandora had "no feelings" about her parents' leaving although she knew she "should." Attending family going-away parties was primarily a pleasant affair for her as she felt good and strong about herself in her new relationship. The separation anxiety she might have encountered, had she not been with Bob, went underground, and Pandora carried her life forward without missing her parents. She discovered that her family had an ambivalent response to Bob, due to his age and the difference in religious–ethnic backgrounds from hers. She tried to ignore her family's responses to Bob and to concentrate on the pleasure of her new relationship.

Although she did not remember many dreams during the early months of dating Bob, the following one (dreamt just after her parents' departure) expresses some of her desire to "fall asleep" in the presence of the separation issues that were coming to the fore. This dream focuses on her sister Emma's wedding (no actual marriage had taken place), which would have felt like a dreadful abandonment to Pandora if it had occurred prior to her meeting a potential marital partner. Because Emma was an alter ego or psychological "sister," we can interpret her wedding also as a fantasized wedding for Pandora herself. If she married Bob, would her family accept him? Was she ready to plunge into a commitment that her father would repudiate and that her siblings would disapprove? Pandora's response is to fall asleep. The dream:

Emma is getting married at a house in the country. People were arriving early and she was not yet dressed. The wedding was to be at 6:00 p.m. and it was now 5:15. My cousin G showed up alone and sat next to me on the couch. Another cousin came too, and helped set up. I fell asleep while waiting on a couch, in the living room, with all the people around.

Mom and Dad were driven in a limousine to a crossroads. It seemed somewhat of a barren place where they were left off, and I realized that they were really gone.

Most of Pandora's ambivalence about Bob as a marriage partner, and her defiance of her Father values and religion, were buried under her conscious desire to make the relationship work.

In their early months, Pandora and Bob encountered several personal crises, including one very traumatic difficulty, which absorbed both our therapy time and her imagination. Off and on during the first 6 months with Bob, Pandora would feel depressed about herself or about her life, but would orient herself more toward trying to "figure out" what was happening with Bob and her. She and Bob decided to live together, although they would do so with no commitment to the future. Bob moved into Pandora's apartment and they set up house on her grounds.

Her parents had left the country in late fall of 1982. In late summer of 1983, she became preoccupied with suspicions and jealousy of what she feared were rivals for her relationship with Bob. Bob had been hired in a beginning position within his profession. His work looked promising for the future. He was working in an office with young women, and occasionally came into contact with a former girlfriend, whom he described as "only a friend." Pandora was at first tolerant, although uneasy, about Bob's contacts with other women, but gradually grew suspicious, especially as she allowed herself to depend on Bob as her only regular companion. In therapy, we emphasized the exaggerated importance she was giving to the relationship as she turned away from her career interests, her previous friendships, and her dissertation.

From the point of view of Pandora's development, she was facing two critial issues in relationship to Bob: differentiation from the Father complex and claiming her own identity as a worthwhile woman with valid interests. The former was represented especially by the differences between Bob and her father. Bob did not have the same values or background as her own father but he was made to carry her Father complex insofar as she believed that he was more intelligent and potentially more successful than she. (Indeed Bob is very bright and promising, but not more than an equal for Pandora intellectually.) She secretly hoped to identify herself with his achievements and career, although he openly told her that he was not ready to get married. More importantly, Bob carried the creative (Hephaestian) animus through his good looks, his suave and controlled style, and his "underground" or punk manner. Pandora became overwhelmed with fears of her inadequacy, especially concerning her weight and appearance. Bob's good looks, in her estimation, seemed superior to her own.

Clearly, we entered more deeply into her basic mistrust of her female goodness as soon as Bob moved into her apartment. Once she possessed her animus-lover, she became fearful about maintaining this union, reactivating low self-esteem and sibling rivalry for the Father. She felt jealous and competitive with any young woman who passed by on the streets.

Much of Pandora's joy in living went underground as she grimly struggled with "what to do about Bob." Should she pursue her suspicious fantasies and check up on him, with the potential of driving him away with her "neediness," or should she contain her fantasies and permit him freedom, in which case he might fly the coop? Developing alongside this preoccupation was a loss of appetite. Almost miraculously she became the svelt woman she had longed to be (especially in the context of competition with the other younger women of her fantasies).

The Hephasestian animus complex grips the woman's desires and pleasures, and reshapes her to be an "evil" seductress of men. The following is a dream near the beginning of Pandora's intense jealousy:

Went to a house with Bob and visited with the woman who owned it. Her apartment in the house was painted a deep red and was decorated with beautiful antiques. I liked it. She was a short woman and looked like a circus freak. I wanted to be touched and she lightly massaged me, but it wasn't enough. I was horny. She started to give Bob a massage and he was genuinely enjoying it. She got sexual responses from him and I was jealous. The massage ended, and we were going to our room—that we had rented in her boarding house. She stood up. Green worms were falling from her feet, grotesque-like.

Hephaestus is, of course, well known for his club feet, his mangled feet. Often Pandora women have dreams about finding the right shoes or of problems with feet. I interpret these generally to mean a problem in "understanding," in getting the right connection to the earth and the female goodness in themselves. In this dream, Pandora associated the dark red color with menstrual blood and pregnancy. The antique furnitue was the sort that she admired and might want to have in her future home.

In terms of the developmental usefulness of this client's Hephaestian animus complex, she was able to see and feel the triumph of her own appearance. Creative strength was actually released in her ability to control the surface of her appearance. A personal connection to appearance and the hidden meaning of it (i.e., that it was designed to trap a man) are missing from consciousness at the Pandora stage, however.

Unfortunately, the feeling of being trapped by the underground animus complex is usually experienced as reinforcement of the dreaded fantasy of a hidden flaw. In this woman's case, her hidden flaw was emptiness. To some extent, the beauty and charm of the circus freak's house are surprisingly powerful components of an interior space. Indeed, Pandora experienced a relief that her underground space was not empty.

After this dream, Pandora began a regression into a more suspicious, at times paranoid, fear that she had been betrayed by Bob. The intensity of this fear moved me to ask about memories of her father possibly betraying her mother. Although she had a vague sense that he might have had some kind of affair, she could not recall any real evidence.

Her jealousy about Bob took a distinct turn for the worse after she returned from a week's trip, with her sister, to the foreign country in which her parents were living. About 2 weeks prior to the trip she had the following dream:

I was at some kind of reunion.

Then I was with my brother and Dad. We were on our way somewhere for a religious holiday. We ended up in a swamp, up to our necks, and a man was sitting in a tree watching us. He said he could help. We got out with his help and he fed us. We were in a forest. The rest of my family showed up then.

I went to an art show gallery of my father's sister, a feminist. She was exhibiting large surreal photos and weavings. My friend was at a table collecting money for the exhibit. She gave me a big hug and wished me Happy New Year.

We interpreted this dream as a sign that she might be moving out of the swampy Father complex and into some new identification with her own creativity.

I did not realize then what intense fears of betrayal were waiting to make their appearance. During her visit with her parents, Pandora felt especially bound to Bob. She even refused to go to a disco with her sister out of a sense of loyalty to him. Her parents disapproved of her relationship with him, and they faced her squarely with the religious, cultural, and age differences to which they objected.

On her return to the United States, she found some evidence that Bob had romantic fantasies about another woman. Pandora was consumed with variations on this theme in her imagination, especially at work and in her dreams. Two themes were prominent during her most intense and tearful suspicion: the betrayal of her trust by Bob, and a reconciliation with Dan. A dream example about Dan depicts the reunion: "Dan was in my dream, and he wanted to get back together. I was so glad to see him." The reconciliation with an internally abandoning animus figure (as with Dan here) can be a signal of further integration of the animus complex as a woman strengthens her self-confidence. I was confused about the conflicting images of reconciliation and betrayal in Pandora's dreams. Typical of the betrayal dreams was the following: "Everything seemed fine with Bob and me, but he went out one night to meet another woman. The next day, he confessed that all along he'd been lying and that he was leaving me for her."

Although she had not yet completely emerged from the troubling anxiety about her inner emptiness, there were many signs, both in her behavior and in her dreams, that she was in the process of discovering her own identity. One thing is certain: The strength of the betrayal images focused her conscious attention on the possibility that the relationship with Bob might end. She has since gradually become able to discern plans for going on with her life without him.

10

Pandora: Transcript, Conclusions, and Epilogue

The language I use in responding to Pandora and my commentary on our dialogue are typical of my therapeutic approach. Although the specific demands of this case and the condition of its public presentation obviously distinguish it from "business as usual," I am satisfied that I have adequately exposed a slice of observational experience from my work as a psychotherapist.

After I had completed the manuscript for both of these chapters, Pandora read over it and made suggestions for some minor changes, all of which I accepted. She continued in therapy with me, and naturally the manuscript became part of our therapy. I was curious as to what effect this exceptional exposure of my own rationale and biases would have on the therapy.

Because of a change in her personal circumstance, Pandora moved away from my city some time after we had collaborated on this report. Consequently, I have included a brief "epilogue" on her case which displays some of the outcome of her therapy and the influence of our collaboration on these chapters.

THERAPY SESSION: ANALYSIS OF AN IDENTITY RELATIONSHIP

At the time of this session, Pandora was working on developing a more adequate self-presentation (persona), one that would enable her to appear to be okay at work and in public situations. She had used thought stopping (thoughts like "What Bob is doing with another woman" and "I am so worthless without him") and had discovered metaphors or images that could provide her with a rational perspective in social situations. A friend had offered an image of just "swimming along" through emotional floods, taking one stroke at a time, so that she would not feel as if she were drowning.

Pandora was functioning at a minimal level of effectiveness at work. She had jeopardized her possibilities for advancement and even for getting good references should she wish to look for another job. She would frequently find herself "just filling up with tears" when her work was tedious, and she would withdraw from the tasks at hand. Similarly she found it difficult to enjoy her former pastimes of reading and music at home. Most of her psychic energy seemed used up in fantasies of betrayal. Her social behavior had changed, and her friends and associates reflected the difference (e.g., "What's wrong with you? You don't seem to be your old self anymore."). Pandora would then become even more frightened, convinced that she would never make it out of the complex. At the same time, she liked her slender appearance and received compliments on her new style of dress, which was more chic and colorful than before.

Prior to this session, I had grown silently impatient with her betrayal fantasies. On one hand, I felt that a real betrayal was certainly possible and that Pandora should be realistically prepared for this. On the other hand, we had interpreted a great deal of the Father complex, with its critical judgments and defeating teasing, and I wanted Pandora to internalize some of these interpretations. Pandora continued to want me to provide interpretations for her and was sometimes enraged that I had not yet cured her.

One Session with Pandora (Session No. 110)

(T: Therapist Young-Eisendrath; P: Pandora)

Commentary

P: I had two dreams, one last night and one over the weekend, that I want to talk about. I've been crying, just filling up, crying, anywhere, tears. It's not every day. Like once a week. Last week it just happened once and then this weekend it was when I was at a friend's house. I just started to cry. Then last night I just started to cry. I tried to call a girlfriend and she wasn't home. So I cried. I stayed in the bedroom for a while, hoping that my tears wouldn't last. I came back out and Bob was there and I guess he sensed

She opens the session by bringing me dreams, something that she knows will be of interest to me. Immediately she tells me that she is not doing well, however, and sets the tone for her position of "not being able."

something was wrong. But I'm so tired of crying and revealing all of this stuff. I guess overall I'm trying to *contain* myself, and take care, but really it's not at a good point especially at *work*. It's like at work I notice a change happens to me. I'm really depressed at work. I mean it's noticeable. Nothing concrete has happened, but I've done concrete things to try to change my work situation. I mean, I think of just quitting and becoming a waitress.

I had previously asked her to "contain" her anxiety and try to direct her energy more toward the tasks around her.

T: So it's focused on your work now.

P: Yeah, it's focused there. And then I think it's a good place to focus it on. The relationship is okay. I mean I'm still a neurotic. I say to him, "If either one of us wants to leave, we should tell the other." (*Laugh.*) "We should definitely talk before we do something." He gives me that assurance. He's been very giving, over the weekend. It's been very comforting.

Here she is referring to her desire for another job and her efforts to find one. Waitressing would be a developmental retreat, an indication of therapeutic "failure."

Unconsciously she may be referring to her ambivalence about her therapy: Either of us should tell the other if we want to leave.

She feels entitled to reassurance.

T: Sounds like you've established more equilibrium.

I am trying to reinforce the positive side of what she has reported.

P: It's . . . honest to God, it's a front. I'd like to really mean it. I did a few weeks ago. But I get to a point when I can't stay in it. Luckily I pull out. I think my ego is somewhat intact because I say "I'm tired." I try to keep it hidden and I think that's a good sign.

She will not let me think about her in terms that sound more capable than what she feels. She wants me to see her pain.

She is in conflict with me about developing a persona, a mode of coping, but she reports that she has been trying.

T: What is the topic—do you know? —which gets focused around the crying?

I focus on the task of understanding too quickly.

P: (*Audible crying.*) I feel lousy about myself (*in a whisper*). It's just I . . . there's nothing I can find good.

This is a repetitive theme that ends in despair.

T: Just feeling worthless.

This emptiness is a constant fear, and the feeling overwhelms her consciousness.

P: Yeah, very much so. And in dreams, it's like I feel: well, Bob and I have been spending a lot of time around each other, and around him I feel *totally* dependent. It's a *horrible* feeling.

T: Feeling like he's the only one who is worthwhile.

This is typical of the identity relationship in women, a retreat behind the worth of the man.

P: Exactly, *exactly*.

T: And his career and his aspirations are more important . . .

P: I don't *have* any of my own right now. And it's driving me up the wall. And intellectually I know what is going on. But emotionally, in my gut, it's killing me. I really feel that I'm being killed off. And I think at times into the dreams I remember, like I am being killed off.

This is a constant experience and one about which she has much assertive conviction.

This is an accurate description of the experience of the complex at this point. She has retreated into animus as Alien Other.

T: Let's hear the dreams.

P: Do you want the one from last night?

T: Yeah, let's start with that one.

P: It really disturbed me. I woke . . . well, what I remembered is: In the dream, I was notified that my father was murdered. He and his brother. That he was murdered. And I was with Emma and it was, it was . . . I was *crushed*. I mean it was a horrible feeling. And the next thing I knew I was up in West City, walking with Emma, and we were in the neighborhood of X.

Unconsciously she is provided with the experience for independence. The dream presents it very boldly as a murder. At the same time, the murder depicts the abandonment she feels by Bob, whom she experiences as alien.

P: I know where I was, on Y street. And I wanna just say that last night I watched the news and there was a murder, there've been a couple of murders up there. There was just a murder of a young woman. And I saw that news, and it really upset me. My sister and I were walking up in that area and we know that Dad was murdered. And we're walking, and we see this Black man

She and Emma are both vulnerable to the Pandora complexes of animus as patriarch or bound Hephaestian creativity.

coming toward us. And it's like, I feel as though we were both over-reacting. We held onto our pocket-books real tight. And I think what happened was that we had great fear in our eyes. And he saw us, and we held onto our pocketbooks, and I don't think he would have done anything except we were really looking at him. I remember he walked by, and I turned to see if he was going to do anything and then he did something. I think it was be-cause I, she and I, antagonized him. To say, "Well, hey, we've got something." "I've got this money in my pocketbook," whatever. So he came after it. Okay? I remember yelling and screaming very *bad* because I brought it on myself. I'm sure he would have walked by had we not overreacted. I think people came down. I think cops came. But I'm not positive. That's all I can remember of the dream. And I woke up and it was still in the mid-dle of the night. I was *upset*. And my heart . . . and I was so glad that Bob was there. And it was just really, ya know, and what upset me a *lot* was that my father was murdered.

T: And did you know how?

P: *No*. It was like cold-blood murder. Brutally.

T: What's been happening with Emma lately?

P: Emma.

T: I mean, have you talked with her lately?

P: Well, she been *very* supportive of *me* lately. She has not been de-manding of me. She's just been there listening to me. I wrote her a letter today saying that I know things have been going on in her

She has been clutching at her self-concept and worth.

Here she reveals that her purse, her female identity, is assumed to be something special in regard to the dark animus figure.

She recognized her own part in instigating the onset of this dis-turbance.

I want to know about her relation-ship, or understanding of this elimi-nation of the Father. She tells me that the complex is alien and that the murder is impersonal.

I wonder if she and her sister have actually been talking about her father.

The report of Emma seems illustra-tive of how Pandora would like the Mother to be.

life, and I don't feel as though I've been terribly *attentive* to her. So I wrote her a note just telling her, basically asking her, for patience and understanding of my situation. And telling her that I *do* know she's going through things and hopefully I'll be able to *be* there for her.

She may feel that she has been attentive to what I want in her therapy, rather than my attending to what *she* wants, which is nurturance.

T: So you were reaching out to say that maybe you were feeling stronger?

Again I try to focus on a positive interpretation of Pandora's self-initiative.

P: (*Emphatically.*) No, *no*, feeling *weak*. But just letting her know that I was feeling weak and appreciating her. And that she might be going through things, but she hasn't been telling me about them because she doesn't want to overload me, telling me stuff. Because I haven't been able to be there for people, I don't think, in a real genuine sense.

Again, Pandora reports that she is not able to fight her complex and focus on others' needs.

T: What does it remind you of, the dream? Does it remind you of anything?

I refocus on understanding. I am thinking of an earlier dream when her purse was snatched by some hoodlums. We interpreted her pocketbook as the focus of her female identity, with its ID cards and money.

P: It reminds me of the other dream when my pocketbook was stolen.

T: Tell me more about that. I was reminded of that too.

P: You know about fighting, for myself, trying to—trying to not let this very destructive part get a hold on me.

Here she returns to the interpretation of the other dream and the task of differentiating from the complex.

T: Here you promoted that yourself because you are really being so, so hypervigilant.

Her constant attention on her inner state is narcissistic.

P: Yeah, yeah. That says to me that's what I've been doing in my relationship somewhat. I feel as though I've been very destructive toward my relationship because I'm so neurotic. I mean it's *ridiculous*. (*Laughs.*)

Here she somewhat acknowledges the narcissism of her preoccupations.

T: If you think of this as a kind of intrapsychic thing.

I want her to look at the intrapsychic meaning, thinking it is more strengthening.

P: Myself?

T: Yeah. The Black man is a negative animus figure. I take it. Someone who would be potentially dangerous, but in the dream is not really that dangerous.

I wanted to emphasize how the alien animus figure might have ignored the situation, if he had not been provoked.

P: Well, ya see, ya know, I've been thinking. I *have* been thinking that this "bad part" is *really* winning out because I haven't been *doing* things, that I know I could do that would be helpful to me.

Here she is disclaiming responsibility for her behavior over the past week.

T: For instance?

P: Ah. (*Pause.*) Trying to be available to people instead of being so self-absorbed. I am really self-absorbed now.

She notes the narcissism that results from absorption in the animus complex.

T: A little more nonchalant maybe. The dream seems to suggest that if you were being a bit more *ordinary*, just by walking by this man and not bringing attention to yourself. . . .

I want to contrast *ordinariness* with the unconsciously assumed specialness.

P: I brought it on.

T: If you think of it as a wound, you are sort of picking at the wound.

I am referring to the attention she gives to her preoccupations.

P: Oh I *am*. (*Relief and crying*.) I can't let go of it. I mean I haven't been *able* to let go of it. So I think to myself: "Oh good, so I'm killing off my father. Great. How come I haven't been released? How come I'm not releasing myself?"

She is honestly struggling here between the pull of the complex and her awareness that she can do something about it.

T: What's your answer to yourself?

P: I think it's got the greatest hold on me right now.

When she can state this emphatically, she feels more certain and stronger.

T: So you keep preoccupied with the fears.

P: That's very true, completely. I'm *very* fearful. I'm fearful of *everything*.

This sounds like a mother explaining her child's behavior.

T: So the dream sort of says that it is the preoccupation with the *fear* that provokes the response from the unconscious, from the negative animus. It is true that the Father complex seems to be rather violently taken away. . . .

I go back to the idea that she could take a more "ordinary" perspective on herself.

This is a somewhat empty interpretation.

P: Well, I don't understand what that means. I mean, more. . . .

T: Right, right, right. What if your father were actually killed like that. . . .

I want to help her get a perspective on the dream, but I am floundering.

P: To be murdered? I would feel very . . . that he was taken unfairly. I mean, if he died of unnatural causes, that would be terribly unfair.

T: How would your life be different?

Finally I ask her to take a perspective.

P: I don't know, don't know. *(Pause.)* I can't imagine, I don't know.

T: If your father died, how would your life be different?

P: I somewhat experience my parents' moving as a death. They're in another country, not here. They're in my conscious, but they're not *here*. I think I would be dealing with the same stuff even if they were here, and even if they were *dead*.

Here she definitely conveys a perspective on the psychological nature of her complexes.

T: Huhuh, *okay*. That gives me a sense that you know what the Father complex is. It's like in the dream, it suggests to me that you are so overly preoccupied with the Father stuff that your dream must take him away violently, stating emphatically that it's *over*. That you need to focus on just who *you* are. How you want to be a person. Your purse, as a symbol of your identity, as we talked about it before, that you need to carry it more confidently, more nonchalantly, without all of this poking at your fears all the time. And I also think the way that

Separation from Father.

the dream states it, you really are still giving your attention to this complex in waking life.

P: I am.

T: That, projecting it onto Bob. Being worried about it at the level of who is going to take care of you. Still, somehow, you haven't recognized that. . . . Uh . . . do you have any other dreams?

I am getting too abstract and want to return to her own images.

P: Yeah. This one happened over the weekend. And all I remember was going to a hospital, into a room and to the right was a Black man sitting on a couch, nicely dressed in his robe. To the left was an old, old man in a bed with white sheets. (*She gestures and describes the room.*) In the corner, behind the old man, was my father's bed. He had fallen out of it, and he was lying on the floor. Sort of, like, dishevelled. Sitting like this in his robe, in a mess. I think Bob went to the hospital with me to visit Dad.

Here the Black man reappears in a very respectable self-presentation. I am struck by the helpfulness of this animus figure, who had been perceived as alien in the last dream. Here he has the persona of respectability that the dreamer needs. The Father is much lower and inferior.

T: So it looks like the Father is really out of it.

P: Those are the *only* dreams I can remember.

T: What does the Black man remind you of?

I wonder if she has noticed the transition of the image.

P: I don't know. He keeps coming up in my dreams. A lot of Black men in my dreams.

T: What do you generally associate with Black men?

P: I don't know. I don't know. I've been involved with Black men.

T: Anything special about Black men?

P: About Black men?

T: Like more sensitive, more tender, more something?

P: No, nothing special. I guess the

A Black man was the first major

only thing with a Black man, was the first man I slept with, rather had intercourse with. A Black man was the first man.

animus projection in a love relationship for Pandora. He was the *first* man.

T: And that was a good experience?

P: Yeah, very good. You know. The Black man in this dream was very presentable. In the other dreams, I was afraid of Black men, terrified. In this dream it was different.

Here she gets to some of the meaning of the integration of a helpful animus.

T: He was the only one who had it together.

P: *Together,* he was the most presentable, right!

T: Can you see yourself, at the moment, having the Black man in you, what he could be. . . .

I am hoping she will find this figure an inner model for allying with her own animus rather than projecting it.

P: I don't know. I keep going back to the *theory,* the blackness. The really scary stuff in me. It's just a real destructive force in me; it's like my own faith in me. The blackness, the darkness. It's the fears that are really eating me up right not. It's destructive, so *active* in me. You know, I mean, at this moment, I feel pretty distant from everything. I could talk to you about any of it.

Here she shifts to the emptiness of her inner self, the fear that she is really only a shell.

T: How would a Black man, if you could imagine it, how would a Black man react to this kind of thing?

P: I guess it would depend on the man. I don't know. It depends on the man.

She's right, of course. I have asked the question too abstractly.

T: How about the guy on the couch?

P: I think he'd be understanding, maybe not understanding to a *depth,* but understanding. Maybe a lot like Bob, I don't think Bob really understands any of this.

She needs to integrate this kind of "ordinary" understanding.

T: I mean if the Black man actually went through this experience of having to see himself as the person on whom to depend, as his own *provider.*

I am pushing the separation–individuation theme here. Again, perhaps I am too abstract.

P: Seeing himself, how would he see himself?

T: The Black man is sort of a marginal person, like women in some ways, in terms of being accepted, getting the right work, and so on.

I try to draw an analogy between her conscious self-concept and the Black man.

P: Huhuh.

T: The Black man on the couch seems quite respectable. How would he handle the situation you're in?

P: Pull himself *together (somewhat sarcastically)* and get out of there, I guess. I don't know, ya know? That's what I want to do. I told you the other week, I don't know what I have to put myself through in order to shed this thing. Because I don't feel in a way I deserve it. What I am doing to myself, *I* don't have that low an opinion of myself, you know what I mean? Because I was functional for a long time and able to get things done and accomplished.

She is rejecting my teachiness and being somewhat cynical about my interpretation.

With this hidden respectability she has somewhat identified with the Black man at the hospital.

T: *Right (emphatically)*.

I want to support this orientation.

P: And I feel as though I deserve to move on, for myself.

T: Yes.

P: But the crying continues, and the self-doubt has grown to be a monster. Got a lot of monsters in me and they *tear* me apart.

She does not want me to forget the strength of the complexes, even for a minute or two.

T: A lot the reason, it seems, that they do is because you pay too much attention to them.

P: I know, I understand that.

T: But you're having a difficult time. . . .

P: Taking them away, putting them back. I mean that I *know*, I can *see* them. They're *cute (laughter)*, they're cute. They have fangs. But I can't get them out.

The cuteness here is interesting because she gets a lot of loving attention for her monsters.

T: Can you stop listening to their voices? Just say "That's not my voice, I won't listen."

This is a typical differentiation interpretation with her.

P: I know, Polly, I've tried. I have *tried*. I've tried to get involved with other things. When things like that happen in the office, I will try to put myself into another space. It doesn't work. I just sorta space out. A woman came into me. . . . We're friendly. She said "What's wrong? You just haven't been yourself lately. You know, you've been quiet, friendly, but not really to yourself. Your smile just doesn't mean much." I had this real vacant look.

Again, she brings me evidence of her inability to struggle against her complexes. She tries to prove that other people see the flaw in her more than I do.

T: Has everyone been noticing a change?

I want to give her a rational context for the idea that not *everyone* sees her vulnerability.

P: No, because I've been keeping to myself. So I think, "Ah." I've been trying to do my acting, but yesterday it just hit me, and I felt like just going out, and I left work early. Bob was also taking the day off, so I went home. I felt my *security*. Polly, I don't know what it is. You know it's like I'm putting everything in. . . . It ought to be in me. I *should* put the focus on me, and I'm not. I know that. I can't bring it into me. I can talk about it, but then when I get to work, to my days. . . . Work is the worst. But wait a second, that's not true. We went away this weekend, and on Sunday it started to erupt . . . because the next day was Monday and work. Bob wasn't there. My friend G said that I was doing just fine, and then, *ffpt*, I just went out. I wasn't there, and I couldn't get back. In the last couple of days, well, right now, the only thing that is keeping me going is my relationship and that's *sick*. That's not good. Lately I've been thinking real bad thoughts.

Here is a good example of how the complex can benefit her, be cute and add to her pleasure.

T: Like what?

P: Well, I don't know how serious it is, but I was thinking, I *was* thinking suicide. Because when I

This is the *bereft of self* experience of a woman in an identity relationship which seems threatened.

get into that vacant space, nothing means anything.

T: I think what you need is some perspective. You get overwhelmed by your mood, by the complex, and you can't *retrieve* a sense of yourself.

P: Well, you know, I told you how I could use that metaphor of swimming that J gave me. But it doesn't hold now. I've been trying to retrieve that. I've been *thinking* that maybe I'm too involved, maybe my therapy is too intense for me. I don't *know*. I don't know. I feel like I'm swimming in it and not getting. . . .

Here she refers to the metaphor that a friend had given her to help her keeping going.

She tells me directly here that I may be causing her distress by pushing her too hard.

T: Not getting a perspective on it. Anything to strengthen your ego would help, would be a thing to do. Do you do any strenuous physical activity?

I'm telling her that only *she* can do this, that I cannot do it for her.

P: I play tennis.

T: With Bob?

P: Yeah, and I play Scrabble. That's been good, though I lost to him last night. I won with my sister-in-law then. You know even these little things matter now.

T: Any other projects going?

P: At work? Well, my job search is underway. I'm starting to make lists. I'm feeling fairly okay about that, about my job. I'm not stagnating right now.

Actually she *was* stagnating in her job.

T: In your job search.

P: Yeah, I'm doing it. I could be doing more but it's okay. I've been reading more. I've been going to bed early to read. I've got the book *August*, and reading it has been good. I wrote that letter to my sister.

I thought this was an interesting choice.

T: Do you find yourself thinking a lot about. . . .

This is not a good intervention because I am inviting more preoccupation with her emptiness.

P: I've been spacing out a lot at work. I find myself staring out the window.

T: What do you think about the future?

Now I try to focus her motivation on a conscious orientation for herself.

P: (*A lot of laughter.*) The *future*? The future!

T: Yeah, like where do you see yourself 5 years from now?

P: That's where I can't get to. I don't know. I don't have that image. Remember when I turned 30? I said that my 30s were going to be reality. Well, that sucks. I think I wanna regress some more and go back to fantasy, my dreams. I wanna go back to that. I'm a lot happier in my fantasies. This reality stuff sucks the big one. I've really been struggling. It's like I have to look at the future and see what I'm doing. Yuck. I was thinking maybe because this weekend I was around a lot of *babies*, and that helped make me more confused. Hmm. The future, the time clock. I was getting pressure from my brother and sister about marriage, the future, what do you want? I said, "I don't know what it is I want." Maybe that added more tears this weekend.

This summarizes our whole session.

Obviously I have touched on some of her feeling of being abandoned by everyone.

T: So when you say 5 years from now. . . .

P: (*Loudly.*) I don't have *any* image. I don't. It's a blank.

T: Seems scary.

P: *Very*, very.

T: 35.

P: Thirty-five and I don't know where I'm gonna be. Thirty-five is a serious time.

The serious time is still in the future, not now.

T: What did you think 3 years ago?

P: When I was in graduate school, I was pretty sure I was gonna be a therapist.

T: Huhuh. What's happened?

P: It's gotten very cloudy right now. I want to do it, but I don't want to do it. Money is a big concern. The *reality* to me is that I'm gonna be on my *own* financially.

This is, I believe, a direct denial of her wish.

T: You don't think you could support yourself.

P: No. Not working in a clinic. I couldn't make decent money.

This is a slight put-down of my profession. Of course, she knows I teach in a college full time.

T: How much would you need?

P: *Need*? Today I said to myself I need new boots. I need shoes and I need boots. Then I said I might need them, but I have boots, I can get by. It's ridiculous: This, you need this, you need that. I don't *need* it. That's nice to have.

She is overtaken by the Mother complex and her anger at not being nurtured.

T: What amount of money would you. . . .

P: (*Loud laughter.*) Well, I don't know. I don't know exactly. I think I'd like to make at least $20–21,000. And to live in a nicer place than I do now, to be able to pay my bills, to be able to go out occasionally. I have not bought a thing for myself in a very long time.

This is a beautiful example of the fusion of the Father complex with the weak Mother complex.

T: So the idea that you have given up becoming a therapist is connected to your desire for financial security.

Her animus projection onto Bob is backed by the Father complex of worldly insecurity.

P: 'Cause my image of working as a therapist in a clinic, we're talking $14–15,000. Maybe in a supervisory position at $18–20,000. I made a call today at a clinic and they said they won't have a position for 2 or 3 years. I could volunteer.

T: I'm thinking that you may have unconsciously killed off this Father

for a reason. There is tension between something like financial
security and the deadness of your
job right now. A lot of the way you
describe your job concerns its deadness for you. Yet it has what you
perceive as security—more than another job would. A job which might
be more creative or interesting to
you. Part of the Father complex is
that feeling of constraint, that you
have to constrain yourself in order
to be safe. You seem to hate working there and want to escape, but
when I raise questions about your
leaving, you say, "Well, this is the
only place that I'm safe."

P: (*Laughter.*) Huhuh.

T: That really baffles me. You call
that *safety*? You're miserable. What
looks like security isn't really safe at
all emotionally. There is no feeling
of satisfaction, being at one with
yourself. And a lot of feeling that
you are a child, that you couldn't
get by without the Father company.
Maybe you won't make as much
money in another job, but you
could become more of a person.
For women, in general—we are
drawn to jobs, like artistic, business,
and human services, which don't
pay much. But then we have to ask
the question about where satisfaction
comes from. Activities are more
satisfying than money. If we take
the masculine dictates about money
as status, if we take those seriously,
then we will never feel that our work
is worthwhile. Then we will always
lose because we will not make as
much money as men. It doesn't
work.

P: No.

T: Even in my work, I wrestle with
this money question all the time.

The dead Father comes into the
picture now.

This is both the Father and
Hephaestian animus, binding up all
her creative energy with fears of
"being lost in the world."

Here I try to expand this idea of
ordinariness in her situation.

I get teachy again.

I want her to identify with my own
choice and my strength as a woman.

I wonder: Is all this struggle worth my effort when I have to struggle so hard financially? I can't afford to charge women very much so I keep my fees down in order to work with women. I realize that feminism is connected with high emotional satisfaction, but lower financial security right now. I want something that fits my own values rather than simply making money. I think you limit yourself emotionally, not thinking creatively about how you could combine clinic work with part-time practice of your own. You could do just *fine*; it wouldn't be spectacular, but you could get into work which really interests you. It might be much more satisfying.

I am trying to offer an alternative to her negative Mother complex.

P: (*Long pause.*) It just scares me what I would have to do. I'm tired of going backwards financially, real tired.

T: Maybe you keep thinking secretly that someday Bob will support you.

Here is the crucial issue.

P: I don't know. That's a real interesting question. Somewhere I say that we are not going to last forever, that this will not be a forever relationship.

T: I'm wondering why would you dream that your father was killed off.

P: I don't understand.

T: Often when dreams give us real violent images of what is missing or gone, it is to turn up the volume, so to speak, on something we are missing or ignoring.

P: So, in my dreams. . . .

T: It's like the dream is saying "There really is no Big Daddy for you after all."

P: But in the dream my father was gone.

T: Maybe you ignore that in waking life. If you trusted in yourself, in your situations, well maybe that Black man would have just walked on by.

P: Walked by, *right*.

T: So I'm thinking that you are still *really* thinking that Bob or someone will provide for you, and that's the reason why you don't make any serious decisions about your future. You're still angry, feeling deserted.

She feels this way about me too.

P: Yeah. That's what preoccupies me, when I'm not with Bob, that he is going to leave me.

T: This wish to be taken care of— it's no longer useful to you. You really need to drop it, your dream says.

P: Why? What makes me keep focusing outside of myself? Why do I keep putting everything out there? Why can't I focus on myself? When I focus on myself, though, I feel so empty. I don't feel much. Right now I don't like to focus on myself. It's like, "oh-oh." That's why I don't focus on myself, because I don't feel much worth in myself.

This is paradoxical, of course, because she projects her own feelings and fears out there so she is still focused on herself.

T: Well, that's your habit, to think you're worthless when there's a struggle. But it's harder to take responsibility. If you left that responsibility up to someone, to your parents, then you wouldn't have to grow up. Eventually, though, you would feel very depressed because you can't turn your back on your development, it's like death.

I want her to see the *death* issue from another side: Her death can be refusal to let go of Father.

P: Yeah.

T: There is no way to get around this. Either you take it on and do it or you suffer from not doing it. It seems easier now to let go, it blends strongly with the feelings of

inferiority. But you also *know*, you
have seen it, that you can be competent. You know the feeling of
success.

P: Yeah, but I don't see now how to
get it back.

In the next session she was able to understand her jealousy about
Bob in a new context. She could see that she had fears about her own
self-worth and attractiveness that were intensely aroused in the relationship with Bob. More importantly, she began to feel some apprehension about their differences: age difference, difference in ethnic and
religious background, and differences in life cycle position (e.g., that
she wants children very soon and he does not). I interpreted this new
ambivalence about Bob as a realistic apprehension from the perspective of Pandora's individuality.

The following dream can be seen as a depiction of the full course
of the relationship between Pandora and Bob since they had moved
in together. The breakthrough imaged in the dream was interpreted
as a breakthrough of the defensive facade (the "strong and teasing
woman") that has held Pandora back from her further development.

Bob and I entered the apartment [Pandora's] building and went up to our apartment. We opened the door, and I could tell someone was in the apartment,
in the bathroom. It was dark. I was terrified, feeling that this man was dead
or a ghost. We were both scared and ran backwards down a flight of stairs,
crashing through the glass doors at the entrance to the building. We got the
police, and I took a bus to the end of the line. There was a bench there. I swam
around in the foam-covered water. I was playful. Another young couple came
up and played around too. It was daytime now. After a lot of waiting around,
I caught another bus back to our apartment. I went up the stairs, still afraid
to go in, and Bob opened the door saying that it was safe to enter. He was
reassuring, but I am still terribly frightened.

Pandora associated the dead person and the backwards flight with
movie scenes in which there is a vaguely defined alien invader. She
talked about the impatience she felt in waiting on the buses, and the
freedom of playing in the foamy water. (Her initial association to foam
was to birth control foam and then to detergent.) She had felt good and
strong in the water. She wondered whether Bob's presence at the end
meant that they would be okay as a couple. I told her that dreams were
not generally predictors of the future, but that the dream seemed to
signal a new kind of safety, possibly within herself, that she could be
at home without fear. With my help, she associated the bathroom to
a childhood dream, told me earlier in therapy: In it a frightening black

witch attacks little Pandora in the bathroom. This bathroom separated her own bedroom from her parents' and sometimes she could hear the noises from their sexual encounters. She often felt the bathroom *both* admitted her to and kept her out of her parents' room. Fearful fantasies about noises had become connected with the bathroom. The presence in the bathroom now prevented her from being comfortable in her apartment with a man. We interpreted the presence as guilt about her fantasied sexual connection to her father.

Because I knew that Bob also had strong abandonment fears (from an early parental death that had not been completely grieved), I guessed that the dark presence in the bathroom represented their shared fears of what was dead, dark, and powerful in their parental complexes. Their crash backward through the facade of the building was interpreted as an intense developmental retreat or regression. Pandora had experienced it as jealousy. She had broken through her old persona of being a strong woman. The public nature of her transportation to the beach, on the bus, was understood as the conventionality (collective form of transportation) of her regressive longings to be taken care of by a male protector. Her arrival at a playful place seemed to symbolize the Mother–Enclosure (La Mer) of the unconscious and pleasurable sexual relationship with Bob (the foam). Returning home, or regaining equilibrium, is a long and tedious process in the dream. She waits on public buses and neither walks nor drives herself. At the end, when she arrives at home, Bob is there to say that their apartment is safe, but Pandora still does not believe it.

The dream is congruent with her felt experience in therapy: Greater belief in her inner security resulted in acknowledgment that she is "safe" within herself, although her feelings of fear remained.

In this case, the patriarchal animus, in the form of the powerful Father complex, was fused with the persona. The creative element of the animus complex was projected. The projection of her creative animus would be caught by boyish *puer aeternus* (or eternally youthful) men whom she saw as sensitive, intelligent, and imaginative. Unfortunately, men whom she romanced tended to be dominated by powerful Mother complexes and hence were vulnerable to depressions, fears of engulfment, suspicion about female power, and desire to flee adult responsibilities. During the early romantic pursuit, Pandora would present herself as the independent, witty, and competitive tease. She appeared to be a *strong* woman. Once she possessed her animus–lover, she would depend on him for most of her creative and emotional stimulation because he *contained* her projected Hephaestian animus. Then she and her lover would lock into an impossible battlefield. She would demand special attention, sometimes as the Father's Daughter and sometimes as the weak Mother, and the man would retreat—either into depression and neediness (Dan) or into silent withdrawal (Bob). The man's retreat would, of course, increase Pandora's demands for attention and activate her fears that she was a weak and empty female who could never manage to bind her man to her faithfully.

At the height of her identity relationship with Bob, Pandora was projecting both the patriarchal and Hephaestian aspects of her animus complex onto Bob and felt bereft of any identity herself. Because she had not achieved an individual identity as a woman, she had to fall back on the Mother complex. The next dream presents more particulars about Pandora's current personality functioning. In the dream she is speaking to the president of her corporation, whom she regularly calls "John," his first name. No other person of her junior status addresses the president with such informality, but she believes that he "likes my kidding around." I have wondered aloud whether Pandora's enactments of being the teasing daughter are actually reinforced in her thoroughly male hierarchial work setting. Her power struggles with male superiors, most prominently with Bill and then with her new boss, have interfered with recognition of her skills. Being casually familiar and teasingly competitive with male authority figures jeopardizes Pandora's possibilities of being taken seriously in many aspects of her work. In the following dream, she takes on John, the president.

I was in a friend's office with John, fighting for a raise. He and I ended up yelling at one another and I told him that he had promised me the raise after 6 months were up. He said that since the new compensation system was in effect, I wouldn't get the raise. It became a yelling match, and he walked out, calling me a name which was an unknown derogatory word that seemed to mean primitive [she associated it to a tribe of pygmies she had seen on TV]. I went back to my office and called Bob. He wasn't home, and he wasn't at work. I wasn't as suspicious as I would be usually. I looked up, and there he was coming to surprise me. He was in his jeans and sneakers. I started to tell him what had happened with John.

The dream accurately depicts the aggressive quality which Pandora sometimes assumed in her fight with male authority figures. She alternates between being the teasing, coaxing Father's Daughter and identifying with the aggressive Father complex. This kind of approach to male superiors may have some sexual appeal, but it does not generally assist Pandora in becoming a respected member of the male group. She can get swamped in feeling like a special outsider, the rare confidante who must be charming and witty. Pandora's challenges to male authority arouse both belittling and competitive responses. "You are so cute when you're mad" is one kind of response she draws while another is simply a refusal to comply with her demands or requests. Although Pandora gets sexualized attention when she acts out her

Father complex, she does not get the results she wants. She has become increasingly frustrated by what she considers to be barriers to her carrying out her own useful and creative endeavors in the work setting. (Many of her "good ideas" are not taken seriously.)

Pandora had begun to acknowledge the value of a more "ordinary" posture at work, with her male superiors. The fact that Bob shows up, at the end of the dream, in his sneakers, might attest to her desire to be loved for her ordinariness rather than for her witty distractions.

I wondered, after the session, if this last dream harkened back to an earlier dream of a 6-month stay in the reformatory, her image of therapy at that time. Perhaps she now felt that Bob or John or someone owed her something for her suffering. Indeed, Pandora does believe that Bob is indebted to her. Because she feels that she has deposited a valuable part of herself into him, she believes that he has entered into a bargain in which he owes her special attention. This is an impossible bargain, of course, because another person can never carry one's own creative development. Bob will always be a disappointment in his inability to give her special attention and to be the exact kind of man she needs. She wants the sensitive and creative man within herself. Releasing her lover to be himself and taking her own interests seriously would be the final outcome of therapy at this stage. Much responsibility will follow from Pandora claiming her interests and pursuing them. Our Pandora has not yet fully encountered this responsibility and she anticipates it ambivalently.

ANALYSIS OF THE CASE

Both the psychodynamic features and the age of this client contributed to how I handled the case. Because this woman was relatively young and still resisting an adult identity as a female, I decided to focus on differentiating the complexes from the personal sense of self. The Mother complex had the form of a dreaded emptiness and weakness. Pandora's preoccupation with jealousy of Bob's fantasized relationships could be understood as her belief that she had nothing to offer in comparison to other women, and that she was nothing in the relationship. The dominating idea about the relationship, then, is that Bob is bound to her out of duty or dependence, not out of love.

I chose to work on defeating her complexes, on differentiating them consciously. My interpretations were focused on reflecting Pandora realistically as a person with competences and weaknesses distinct from the parental complexes and from the unrealized, projected creative animus. As a conscious process of separation and differentiation, this tends to undermine the complexes rather than explore them. That is, the focus of analytic interpretation is more often on the reductive, historical side and more often distinguishing between the woman and her fantasies. Consequently, the client can experience the therapist as fighting with her about the reality of her experience. The client claims these monsters are real, and the therapist explains them away.

Furthermore, the therapeutic alliance with the Pandora client is often threatened by projection of the negative Mother complex. If the female authority figure is not to be trusted, based on the client's internal dynamics, then the female therapist is not to be trusted. The anger awakened within the therapeutic field between client and therapist can be used by each one to strengthen the fight against the complexes, and to clarify the boundaries between the client and therapist, between the personal and archetypal. For example, Pandora's expression of anger at me was used to show her that I was strong enough to take anger and criticism, that I would recover the creative, therapeutic process in the face of her anger. Thus I could be distinguished from the weak, empty Mother. I could also be distinguished from the aggressive, competitive Father if I did not return the anger or simply fight. Finally, because her anger could be explored and understood in therapy, it was taken seriously and not as a part of a manipulative game, demonstrating that Pandora could be seriously responsible for her anger and not just *cute* when she was mad.

By approaching the analytic task as differentiation from the parental and animus complexes, I am setting myself up for battle and ambivalence. On my side I have techniques, empathy, and humor, as well as my faith in the developmental process of psychotherapy (especially in the imaginative capacity of dreaming). On their side, the complexes have strong emotions, images, and habits, which are familiar to both the client and to me. I must be capable constantly of differentiating my own strategies and perspective from the fantasized elements of the complexes. At the same time, I must be open to listening to the complexes as they are personified in dreams and enacted in the moment, to discover what they are saying. This is a task of acuity and responsibility, which can be quite exhausting and thankless. The effective female therapist, with a Pandora client, will ultimately experience the good work of therapy as the client's taking credit for the work that was done as she departs. Just as the good-enough mother to the teenage daughter will be rejected, so will the good-enough therapist. Not that the client will be unappreciative, but the client should feel that she has achieved her own perspective and has made her own decisions.

In this case, the intensity of the identity relationship and the age of my client contributed to my impatience at times, and to my fears that perhaps I had understood this client to be more capable than she really was. I constantly had to return to her realistic competence and recall her achievements when I would temporarily lose faith in my understanding of the dynamics. Ultimately, I have discovered Pandora's ability to gain strength in the face of weakness, and to provide a net to catch herself. The net is made of realistic strengths, of useful metaphors and images, and of learned self-control. Eventually she will have enough sense of self to look inward at her own female nature and to take seriously her desires for an individually useful and creative life.

EPILOGUE

The narrative of the Pandora case was completed in early 1984. After we finished working on the manuscript and returned to a more "normal" atmosphere, Pandora discovered that Bob had indeed been making alliances with another woman. With my support, Pandora confronted him with her terms for a monogamous commitment. Bob was fearful and eventually moved out of her apartment. He began to date other women, but periodically he would return to Pandora, sometimes late at night, and gain admittance to intimacy with her.

Here is a dream that Pandora brought to therapy after Bob moved out:

Bob and I were walking back home. He had just worked out (at a gym) and I had my work clothes on. My purse was snatched by two Black guys and I screamed. Bob took off and pursued one. The other guy turned around and shot me in the upper, inner, right thigh. I fell to the ground and the police and ambulance came. The next thing I knew I was on the floor in the hospital. The doctor or attendant was also there. He was a light-skinned Black man. He eventually left the room, and I wondered why I wasn't on an examination table. I thought the wound was small, looked like the size of a BB pellet puncture. I wondered if I would get visitors at the hospital.

Pandora and I interpreted this dream in terms of her desire to be rescued by Bob from the aggression of her own animus. Bob is imaged as powerful and muscular, and Pandora has once again lost her purse to the darker male within. The wound seemed trivial to her, even in the dream. Her focus was more on the self-pity and her desire for attention (visitors). Why the inner right thigh? Pandora thought her legs were her "best feature," and she said that a wound in her thigh might scar her beauty.

During this period of early separation from Bob, Pandora repeatedly returned to her fears of growing old and ugly. She assumed that Bob's attractions were for younger women and she could not (refused to) validate her own worth and interest.

Gradually, into the beginning of March, Pandora began to feel herself a separate person from Bob. She found her work increasingly more interesting and she began to conceive of herself as a "free woman." Additionally, her sisters both helped her put a more objective light on Bob. They counseled her to let go of him because of religious, ethnic, and age differences between them. I focused much more strongly on the analytical work of our therapy and backed away from a crisis orientation, taken during the breakup period. Still, Bob and Pandora continued their nighttime alliances, although less frequently.

The following dream, reported about a month after the preceding one, marked a turning point toward the greater integration of animus. This dream is an example of the sort of dream which signals an awakening of Pandora's "curiosity" in the final phase of therapeutic work with such a client.

I was back in my childhood town. The whole family was gathered in an apartment on top of a small restaurant. I went out for a walk and discovered in the street some jewelry. Three Seiko watches, diamonds, rubies, bracelets, and necklaces. I scooped up the jewels and took them home. I wanted to show my family what I found, but I thought that some of the strangers who were visiting were "suspect." So my older sister persuaded me to show the jewels, but I was paranoid, wondering if some thief might be watching, even planning to blackmail me.

Pandora began to realize that the thief, the dark animus who would "snatch" her identity and self-worth, was a part of her own paranoia. Although she had recognized this aspect of her animus influence previously, she now began to take on responsibly a desire to change her attitude. Over the next several months, she worked to see herself in a more positive light: connecting up to new friends (including some men), inquiring about her dissertation status at the university, and making several proposals at work.

During this time, Bob was making a decision to move to another city and asked Pandora if she would consider going with him. He was reevaluating his love for her and decided that he didn't want to lose the "best relationship he had ever had." Although Pandora was strongly tempted, she realized that an impulsive move would leave her without a job and without a network of friends.

Bob moved and Pandora was left to live alone. Just before his move, she reported the following dream:

I met up with a 50-year-old woman whom Bob was having an affair with. I was incredibly upset and confronted him about her. In a cocky manner, he told me he was screwing not only her but women from 13 to 50 years old. The hurt of betrayal was severe and I walked out on him. My heart was pounding.

We both congratulated her that she was beginning to integrate, even into her dream self, the reality of some of Bob's limitations. In terms of Pandora's associations to the ages of the women, she talked about her own awareness of her father's potential infidelities to her mother (when she was about 13 and her mother was about 50). Obviously the alliance between the weak Mother and the aggressive, betraying Father was beginning to break down as Pandora "walked out" on the affairs.

Pandora's self-confidence increased. She appeared to be feeling (in the separation from Bob) the expectable grieving process: She began to be enraged with him. She could (for the first time) see how much he had taken advantage of her and how limited he had been in his ability to share in her development. She spent several therapy sessions simply reviewing for me the ways in which she now saw her earlier feelings about Bob as "fantasy" and "projection." Several times when Bob appeared at her doorstep now, she had turned him away. She told me with surprise, "He even looks different to me! I can't believe that I thought he was so handsome and special; he's a fairly ordinary-looking guy." We were both appreciative of the following dream which seems to indicate the discovery of the Black-man animus as a positive influence.

I met Michael Jackson as he was on tour. I got to help with the tour and to see him "live in concert." He came by my apartment (which was above a store) and his hair was in a "natural." He was regular looking. We had to be at the concert hall by 3 p.m. We left and I realized that I had forgotten his whistle (an important symbol). I got off the bus and ran home to get it.

She mentioned how "important" she had felt being in this alliance with Michael Jackson. We associated the concert with her therapy since it also occurred at 3 p.m. We talked about my desire for her to be "in concert" with her animus, and she said she finally understood what I was talking about. I introduced the possibility, however, that she felt like she was "serving" the specialness of others, for Bob, for MJ in the dream—and even for me (as she had offered herself as the subject of these chapters).

This opened up the topic of her being the "youngest child" and feeling herself to be generally inferior to all of the "others." We reviewed the fact that Pandora was the best educated, most highly achieving member of her family. We talked about how easily this reality slipped away.

We also talked about the fact that I had idealized Pandora and she had idealized me. Together we were vulnerable to forming a "protective covering" of idealization in our relationship. I had often been reluctant to say how impatient, even angry, I had become in dealing with Pandora's refusal to take back her animus projections onto Bob. She, on the other hand, had not expressed her frustration at me at times when she had felt it, especially involving the case history. She had felt I was "creating" her in a way which suited *my* needs in the case, reducing some of her achievements and emphasizing her jealousies about Bob.

This kind of introduction led us to work on the Mother complex. Pandora spent the last several months, before leaving therapy, confronting both her aggression and her despair about Mother. During this time, her mother and father spent a month visiting their children, and Pandora was able to speak openly and to set boundaries on her mother's incessant complaining. Pandora began to see her mother as a person. In the midst of this insight, she had the following dream:

I went to Mom, who was in an asylum. She was there for a week of rest and evaluation. I was terribly upset to see her in this condition, but knew that she was finally being cared for. There was much more to the dream that I can't recall. Bob was there too.

Although Pandora was not able to express any immediate tenderness toward her mother, she was able to sense the difference between her mother and herself. Aware now that she was not bereft of self as her mother had been, Pandora was increasingly able to remember her own greater intellectual, social, and financial independence.

Simultaneous with much of this working-through of the Mother complex, Bob began to approach Pandora again—this time with a marriage proposal. Throughout several months of apparently reasonable negotiations, Bob and Pandora became engaged.

Finally, Pandora left Philadelphia to share an apartment with Bob. They chose a place together, near a university where Pandora could complete some additional courses, a place they both thought was a "fair compromise" in terms of personal inconveniences. When Pandora decided to make the move, she recommitted herself to finishing her graduate studies.

In our final sessions, we encountered many elements of our idealization of each other. Most prominent were her anger that therapy was "not yet finished" and my worry that her "specialness" in treatment with me might influence her negatively in making another treatment alliance. I believe that we adequately worked through the distortions of these concerns while acknowledging the reality of the risks we had taken. Pandora had made a substantial developmental transition in the last phase of our therapy. Through the integration of the weak Mother complex, she seemed to be entering the Psyche Stage in which an internalization of "good-enough" fathering permits a woman to enter courageously into her authentic identity.

11

Heroic Complex and the Death Marriage: A Case of Transforming Childhood Sexual Abuse

When Psyche first entered therapy with Wiedemann, she had much in common with Pandora. She was articulate, attractive, and intelligent, a woman of 35 entering her midlife phase. She had adapted to a rather traditional feminine model for gender identity—she was slender and fashionable, and she affected a wide-eyed innocence that made her seem at once vulnerable and trusting. Her features were strikingly beautiful, and she obviously knew how to use makeup to her best advantage. For all this, however, she struck one immediately as a woman in trouble. Her expression was tense, furtive, almost grim. Her shoulders looked stiff and slightly hunched; her chest, caved in. She constantly raised her hand to her mouth as she spoke, making it, at times, difficult to understand her and strongly suggesting a personality plagued by fear, confusion, guilt, and ambivalence. Yet, she seemed courageous and determined in the way she clearly stated her reason for coming to therapy. Her life, as she described it, was "falling apart at the seams," and she couldn't understand the reasons. She had come to "find some answers."

PERSONAL HISTORY

Unlike Pandora, Psyche had actualized an identity relationship with a man. Eight years before, she had married a successful young lawyer, Taylor, onto whom she clearly had projected the attributes of her Father complex: intelligence, power, and worldly success. At the time, she now recalled, her marriage had seemed like the greatest triumph of her life:

My family loved him, I loved him . . . it was wonderful. I mean, *he* was wonderful. He was only 28, and he already had this huge law practice, and believe me, I wasn't the only one interested in him at the time. In fact (*Psyche laughed nervously at this point.*) I'm still not certain why he chose me. But I don't care—I mean I didn't care. Not then, at least. I was a dental hygienist. You don't expect to latch onto a man like Taylor when you're cleaning teeth for a living. When he asked me to marry him, I felt as if I had just won the lottery.

When Psyche married Taylor, she was blindly infatuated by his power and promise. But her future did not work out as smoothly as she had hoped.

Her first disappointment had come as a shock when she realized that despite determined efforts, she couldn't conceive a child. All during the first 4 years of her marriage, she had felt humiliated and confused by her apparent "gynecological problems." Through a round of doctor visits and extensive advice from friends and family, Psyche had finally established a routine of temperature taking and scheduling sex to adapt to an irregular fertility cycle. By the time she finally became pregnant, Psyche had grown discouraged and felt weary of "sex on demand." That was when she began to describe herself as "sexually frigid." She confessed to feelings of "disgust" and shame at her sexual retreat from Taylor. Then, just after the birth of her daughter, Reid, she had another shock. She discovered that Taylor was having an affair with his secretary—an affair that had apparently been going on for 2 years. Yet, even with evidence of the affair before her eyes, she moved neither to separate from him nor to confront the difficulties of their situation. Now, after years of depression and shame, Psyche was finally willing to "find out what had happened" in her marriage to Taylor. At the same time, she firmly decided to leave him forever.

Her move to sue for divorce was the "death marriage," her leap into darkness, searching for a confrontation with herself. The decision to divorce had been extraordinarily difficult for Psyche because she had always been a "good girl" and had tried hard to approximate the ideals of femininity and nurturance that she believed to be embodied in her mother. That she was now divorcing the man whom she had once revered and was entering actively into single parenting of her young child seemed to Psyche to be undeniable evidence of her "failure" as a woman and a daughter. Moreover, she was "afraid of the responsibility" of single parenting and concerned about managing her finances. More significantly, she was "outraged" at the betrayal and "confused" about how her wonderful romance with Taylor had degenerated into hostility and deception.

From a deficit perspective, Psyche met many of the criteria for Histrionic Personality Disorder in that she displayed what is often described as a "dramatic and seductive" style of femininity. She reported feelings of profound fear and confusion in the presence of demands from authoritative men such as Taylor, her boss, and her father.

Over the course of treatment in the first year, Psyche gradually recovered repressed memories of sexual abuse. In the second and third years she was able to translate these memories and their associated feelings into a new sense of herself. When she recognized that she had endured both a traumatic abuse and its remembrance without collapse, Psyche felt an inner strength and courage which were remarkable.

In the first year I saw Psyche twice weekly in analytic therapy. In the second and third years, we met weekly. In the fourth year, we met twice monthly, and in the fifth and sixth years, I saw her about four times per year.

In terms of the overall development of Psyche's personality throughout the 6 years I have seen her, I would assess her as moving from Loevinger's Self-Aware Stage to the Individualistic Stage of ego development. When she entered therapy, she had adapted to a Pandora orientation but had made a determined commitment to understanding why her marriage had failed. Her desire to be approved, to conform, and the degree to which she valued niceness and helpfulness— characteristic of the Conformist Stage—initially seemed to contrast with her determination to understand herself and her motives. At the time of this writing, Psyche clearly exemplifies an Individualistic orientation, cherishing both her autonomy and her relationships with her second husband and daughter. She has accepted the fact that conflict and ambivalence are intrinsic to human relationships and has been able to see how these contribute to growth. Obviously, Psyche has developed substantially, both cognitively and interpersonally, during the time I have known her. In the following account, I trace this development.

PHASE ONE: DIFFERENTIATION OF ANIMUS
AND NEGATIVE MOTHER COMPLEXES

The initial treatment phase provoked recollections of Psyche's most troubling repressed memories. Hence her therapy had a somewhat different character from some other women at this stage of development. Significantly, her parental complexes and animus were bound together in such a way that her adaptation could not have continued without a rigid inhibition of her personality development.

Psyche actively surrendered herself to treatment and to a confrontation with her own motivations, needs, and desires. Her intelligence and cognitive complexity, as well as her interpersonal resources and career competences, made her an excellent candidate for analytic treatment. Our rapport developed rapidly as Psyche initially saw that her enclosure in the Father complex (Pandora adaptation) had resulted in a limited and repetitive life structure. She longed for experiences of her own authentic goodness and repeatedly complained that she had permitted Taylor to direct her life in much the same way her parents had.

In the second month of treatment, Psyche reported the following dream, accompanied by an expressed fear that she was "going crazy."

I'm looking in a mirror, like you look at yourself first thing in the morning trying to get ready to go somewhere. My hair has alfalfa sprouts growing in it, and as I watch, it's getting bigger and bigger. I try and get rid of some of it and it only makes it grow more. Finally I decide, well hell, I'll just have to leave it because I'm running so late. I'm not at all upset—am only amused.

Although her attitude of "amusement" in the dream suggests a denial of the strangeness of what is coming out of her head, Psyche reported in therapy that she was worried about what might be uncovered as we continued. I too was concerned because I sensed a serious depression just beneath her defenses. I doubled her sessions.

Shortly thereafter, Psyche began to tell me about "Uncle." Psyche's family had lived next door to her father's sister during 3 years of Psyche's childhood, from age 5 to 8. The sister's husband became Psyche's caretaker when Psyche's mother was hospitalized for some surgery and Psyche was left in his charge. Psyche had distinctly painful feelings about Uncle, which she associated initially with his sudden, untimely death after her aunt divorced him in later years. I wondered about her painful feelings and pressed her to remember more.

In place of memories, Psyche developed physical symptoms. She had chest pains and nausea both within and outside of therapy sessions. Entries in her daily journal read as follows:

I'm in my hell hole tonight. I can't get out. My chest hurts and I can't stop crying. I can't eat but thank God I'm not nauseated. I feel as if I'm breaking apart. I'm so angry and sad and scared. I'm not sure I can go through with this. What am I going to do? I need somebody to hold me and love me, and I can't do it for myself.

A stormy and difficult year of therapy ensued in which I often worried that Psyche would literally fall apart and become unable to work or care for her child. But Psyche's willingness and courage were firmly backed by her ego adaptation as she was able to come in and out of therapy twice a week, and continue to fulfill her daily responsibilities.

Remembering the sights, sounds, and smells of the involvement with Uncle was a deeply disturbing experience for both of us. Psyche would sit on the floor by my knees (by her choice, as she had sat on the floor with Uncle) and relive the scenes: the linoleum floor, the yellow light from the lamp, the terror she felt as he cornered her and forced her to perform fellatio. These scenes, in fact, were only the beginning. As she continued to recount her stories, she recalled also his words and his dictates to her. The following are excerpts from a tape of a therapy session about midway through the first year:

His bed-couch. My head pushing against the back of it. It hurts so much. Wrinkled sheets. Very dark. No one here but him. I hate him!

Penis, corners, dirty, where's the door? I am gagging, choking, feeling smothered. It feels good, but it hurts and I am so ashamed.

He has to put me on the table. I have to sit on a pottie chair he built for me. He says there are so many poisons inside me. He says it's so evil and hot in there. He has to stuff ice cubes inside to cool it down. He has to clean it out with cotton and alcohol because it's so dirty in there. Then he forces me to take his penis in my mouth. He tells me to lick it and the smell is awful! Then he rapes me. He tells me that it is all my fault. If I didn't have so much evil in me, this wouldn't happen. He has to clean me out again. I am shaking and quivering, so cold. He draws red marks around my nipples and puts lipstick on my mouth. I feel so ashamed.

Psyche and I were able to understand much about her feelings of shame, the unintentional covering of her mouth, her choice of dental hygiene as a profession, and her fear of men from these memories.

As she recovered the memories more directly, Psyche was burdened with enormous feelings of guilt. She remembered that she had told her mother about the sexual abuse when she was 8. Her parents confronted her aunt and uncle. It was this confrontation that resulted in the aunt's divorcing the uncle. Soon after, her uncle had died of a heart attack, alone in the streets. Psyche unconsciously took responsibility for his death, accepting her later difficulties with Taylor as atonement for her guilt.

Gradually, another side to her story emerged. Fundamentally, Psyche blamed her mother for having abandoned her to the torture of her uncle. Self-inflicted punishments connected to guilt over her uncle's death had functioned also to inhibit her aggression against her mother. In her dreams she began to encounter aggression more directly, portrayed as attacking a weak or confused Mother complex, as in the following.

Mother is reaching out to me to keep me from falling—into the water, I think. I have a broom in my hands and every time she reaches out, I hit her hand with the broom. I am very calm and unfeeling about this.

A dream reported two sessions later shows a new attitude developing.

Mother and I are riding in a car on a road that seems to always move up. I say something to her, some feeling of some kind. She says "No, you are wrong to feel that way. You should feel another way." I say that she has no control over my feelings and that what she does in making these judgments is to force me away from her. She is terribly hurt. I don't feel that I should amend my statement or apologize. I'm driving. We stop at a house that sells hamburgers. They are shaped like the road we've been driving on. We climb up the stairs and start on the same road again, over and over. When we get to the top, Mother is so exhausted that I have to carry her. Our food is ready. When we get ready to leave the cashier says, "Use the door over there. It goes directly into the street. It's not necessary to climb so many steps."

Psyche's relationship with her mother actually changed as Psyche began to be more dominant in stating her needs. She refused to let her mother spoil her accomplishments by speaking of them in an envious or depressed way. Psyche recognized that nurturing (the hamburgers) between her and her mother had been mightily disrupted by repression and suppression of their actual desires and feelings. With this, she was able to let go of some of the overprotective attitude she had felt toward her mother, principally a result of her hidden shame and rage.

The emotional shift from fusion to differentiation of the animus and parental complexes is depicted in the images and actions of the next dream. Psyche was beginning to separate out an authentic sense of herself from intrusions of her complexes.

I have stolen something. It's a statue of a nude man (white alabaster) and woman, arms and legs wrapped around each other. They're standing, cheeks touching, tears running down their faces. They're comforting each other. They're holding each other in real need. I am running—trying not to drop it! It's so very heavy. I arrive at some sort of boat dock where a boat is waiting. There are three persons waiting in the boat; an old woman (leathery face—75, brown rags, blue apron, and chuckling), a woman in the lavender shawl (Psyche's age), and a demon man, metamorphized into someone more human. I am afraid and tired, and I get in the boat. I hand the statue to them and they lay it in a bed of sorts and cover it with green army blankets. The demon (human body with tail, not frightening, gentle) lifts me into the boat and kisses me on top of the head. The old woman is driving the motor boat and we take off down a canal-like body of water. The houses on either side are large, multistoried dwellings that are directly against the water. The color is like red-washed adobe. The sun is shining on them (green shutters and tall roof) but not on the water. We are *traveling* (feels neat—not out of control) *very fast*. I can feel the wind and the water spraying in my face.

Psyche associated the alabaster statue with abuse, a rather compassionate version of the enmeshed attitudes of aggression and attachment she had encountered in relating to Uncle. She has stolen the statue and it is quite heavy; that is, this depiction of the abuse is not yet quite her own. (It is perhaps stolen from the therapist.) The demon and old lady seem to be personifications of Father and Mother complexes currently alive in Psyche. Although the old woman is driving (therapist leading the way), Psyche is openly trusting the journey ("Feels neat—not out of control"). This trust was a signal of a new level of work in her treatment, a capacity to encounter her abandonment depression and its consequences in her internal victimization.

Psyche reported that she felt "a great weight has been lifted." She said further, "It's as if I don't have to punish myself anymore. It's like I've been living in the dark in some private sort of hell and now I can come out and not feel so terrified. I still feel scared of all the hours I'm going to be alone. . . . I feel as if I am recuperating from a long illness."

In the first phase of Psyche's therapy, she and I worked to construct a new attitude toward herself—a way of looking at her life and her work not burdened by shame and guilt. We set the stage for discovery of her self-interests, her motivations for working and forming relationships.

For some women in the Psyche stage of development, we can reach this first goal of therapy rather quickly through analysis. For this client, there was a profound regression, in the service of further development, during which my role was supportive and clarifying rather than primarily analytical.

PHASE TWO: INTEGRATION OF HEROIC ANIMUS AND NEGATIVE MOTHER COMPLEXES

Over the first year of therapy with Psyche, I was impressed by a gradual transformation of both her self-presentation (persona) and her feeling life. Apparently, the repression and alien impulses of the rapist animus, intermingled with an unexamined and largely projected Father complex, had contributed to her rigidly feminine persona. Psyche's emotional expressiveness changed, and she appeared less inhibited in declaring her competence and authority. She was able to talk about her feeling life in a richer, metaphorical way and to maintain an analytic attitude toward her complexes. The self-consciousness, embarrassment, and naive attitude melted away and were replaced by a more decisive manner.

During this second phase, Psyche saw me as a "model" of what she would like to become. She wanted to be a mother who had a vital relationship to a man while she was involved in a career that she enjoyed and in which she could be creative. Because she experienced her Mother as someone who could not empathize with her independent (different) experiences, Psyche was apprehensive about my ability to sustain her through the process of developing an independent life. Would I disapprove of her choices? Would she have to please me by becoming "a successful career woman" as she had tried to be a perfect mother?

Many dreams of the negative Mother complex emerged as we worked to imagine her best potentials for the future. I often felt tested, as if she were an ambivalent adolescent daughter who both wanted my approval and wanted independence from my opinion.

Responsibility for her own needs and interests was the conscious focus of our work. Psyche made a decision to pursue graduate education—a master's and a doctorate degree in education. This decision was the product of much struggle and differentiation both from me and from Mother. In her daily life, this decision meant juggling long working hours with 45-minute drives back and forth to the university, mothering her child, and completing classwork.

The conflicts aroused by these competing activities and roles continued to focus on perfectionism. Psyche wanted to be all things to all people, and her desires exhausted her. Curiously, as Psyche entered the "treadmill" existence of responsible life, she had several dreams which presented her as traveling through a spiral, reminiscent of Ariadne's trip into the labyrinth. These dreams depict a kind of anxiety felt by a Conscientious person who idealizes responsibility and seeks perfect fulfillment in every aspect of life. The following dream is illustrative of the anxiety provoked by the heroic animus when it is not integrated.

Am taking a psych class in humanistic health care under Dr. G (my mentor). I'm running very late and feel it is so imperative that I get to class on time since it's the first class. Traffic is a real problem and class has begun when I arrive. There is an assignment on the board that we are to plot a graph from the given information in order that we may better understand the lecture. My rendition is as follows:

Under the graph there is a picture of a woman, and there are minute holes in the paper in some random manner. The woman is lovely, my age, eyes shut, mouth open.

Dr. Grant walks in and begins to speak. A woman in the back of the room raises her hand. She is around 50, has dark hair, wears tortoise shell glasses, and has on a plaid skirt and red sweater. She says, "We've been doing experiments on chickens and have reached the conclusion that when asked a question, they will only respond when the question is prepared by using their name to get their attention." I say, "That sounds like bullshit to me. People are not that selfish. They do care about what happens to you. Oh, dear God, please let someone be listening to me. I need help. I know where I'm going but I don't want to do it by myself. Can't you see that from my graph."

We associated the woman wearing tortoise shell glasses to an authoritative woman professor in her life. The woman seems to present a scientific attitude, but she speaks nonsense. Psyche often regressed into the victimlike stance of a helpless little girl (Persephone underground) in the presence of an authoritative person. Although she is aggressively confrontive ("That sounds like bullshit to me."), she also retreats into a passive helplessness reminiscent of her older adaptation as Pandora.

She and I repeatedly encountered her Great Mother idealizations of me accompanied by her puzzled hurt when I did not fulfill her expectations. Similarly, she idealized a new male friend, Tom, whom she found "very exciting." She met Tom, a professor of architecture, during her second year in therapy. Tom was 42, the father of two adolescent children, and divorced from his wife of 14 years, whom he described as "frightfully demanding." By Psyche's report, Tom was worried about her "demands and clutching." I confronted Psyche with the possibility that her idealizing of Tom and me were narcissistic wishes for us to meet her needs perfectly. She had projected onto Tom an ideal heroism that he could never meet—"very sensitive and compassionate" and "always responsible for his children."

Her desire to please me and to be "a very good client" was congruent with our work, but was a defense against being aware of her own self-interest. The next dream is typical of many in which Psyche imagined that *I* (as the longed-for positive Mother) was at the center of her personality.

I'm at a pavillion with different levels, and the moon is shining. There are Chinese lanterns and the night air smells incredible, like redwood and damp leaves. It's very peaceful. I'm with a man and a woman who is his wife, and I'm his mistress. He's very gentle and solicitous. The man says, "I want you to meet someone." He took me to an Indian woman in a shawl with a gray bun of hair sitting on a low table. She's doing something with her hands. He says, "This is your mother." She smiles, and I walk over and sit down. The old woman helps me put a rock back together that keeps breaking up. The Indian woman feels accepting, easy, nonquestioning; no pressure, she's serene.

The rock crumbles, and crumbles, and I'm alone on a large rock in the water. It's a glistening night and the moon is reflecting on the water, and suddenly, the rock fuses back together.

The fusing of the rock is a very hopeful image, but the power of integration is still contained within the positive Mother. The desire for restoration to a "perfect wholeness" is a regressive desire that is often intensely experienced by children who have been abused. As long as Psyche held this desire concretely, she would demand of herself and of the world a perfect life, something obviously unachievable.

At the university, she found herself idealizing one of her professors and projecting onto him the heroic animus. The projection of heroism onto professors is a typical infatuation with the heroic animus.

Her next dream reveals the wish to possess the supplies of the idealized Mother (presented as a rich collection of fabrics which she associated to my clothes and office) allied with her new infatuation. Anxiety about meeting masculine standards ("on a merry-go-round") leads to an impulse to fall in love with her male professor.

I am sitting in the medical school library reading when suddenly the room begins to spin and it feels as if I'm on a merry-go-round. I reach for something but it's just out of my grasp. Finally I reach it and am able to stop the room from spinning. The handle that I grab has a set of keys attached to it. I pull them off the handle and walk to a very large antique glass-front cabinet. I put the key in the lock and open the large doors. There are clothes hanging in there—beautiful blues, grays, and lavenders—silk, lace, linen, heavy cotton, every fabric imaginable. I begin to try on the clothes, oblivious to other people sitting in the library. They are all so beautiful and feel so good that I begin to stack them next to the chair I'd been sitting in, thinking that I'll take them all. Dr. S walks over and says, "You can't take all those." Dr. G (my mentor) walks up behind me and places his hands on my shoulders and says, "Oh yes she can. This is a special event and it's important that she do so." I turn to him and put my arms around his neck and kiss his cheek and say, "I love you, Allen."

We interpreted the keys as her aggression, necessary to unlock the potential of her new possibilities at the university, as distinct from her narcissistic wishes to simply lay claim to supplies which were not hers.

At the time of this dream, Psyche was faulting Tom for not being able to "help out" enough with her situation due to his busy schedule. Tom began to retreat, fearing "engulfment," and Psyche abruptly ended their relationship. She had become intolerant of the limitations of his situation compared to the ideals of her heroic animus. In the dream, Dr. G promises her all the "riches," saying that she can simply have them.

For Psyche especially there was confusion between her desire for intimate support from men and her sexual desire At this point, she was still vulnerable to enacting her desire for support as a sexual arrangement. Such enactments of the Father complex are frequently distressing by-products of women's negotiations with male authorities (e.g., administrators and professors) in which men are also vulnerable to seductive and manipulative arrangements with subordinate females. In the following dream, Psyche is "about her father's business."

I'm there, and Dr. G (head of department) and lots of people from school are here. Dr. G (Allen) and I are in bed together.

It's quiet and we're talking. I touch him and we start to make love. Phone rings and it's mother. It's 2 a.m. She's crying and says, "I'm terribly sick—will you come?" I tell him I have to go to Mother but I'll be back. Allen gives me a gold key. I go to Mother and she's not really sick and I'm so angry. I say, "Why would you do this?" And she says, "Because I need you and you don't need me." I go back, and I've lost the keys. Mother has them. I go back and have to physically yank them away. Back in bed with Allen and she calls again, I say, "Don't call me. I have to be about my father's business."

Psyche was forced to confront her own identification with the abusive and abandoning Father. She could repeat the "sins of the father" in relating to the important men in her life. The old Mother in the dream is angered by the heroic embrace. She appears as a helpful, irritating force, a reminder of Psyche's actual need to become aware of her shameful and harmful impulses. In claiming her potential to be an abusing Father and a negative Mother, Psyche connected her childish expectations to her assumptions of the power of sexual favors with men and her wish that Mother would save her from enacting them.

This recognition brought feelings of loss and depression. She must now fully claim to be an adult. No longer could she simply wish to be cared for or approved by a powerful other. These functions reside within her own personality and she must set aside her magical thinking in favor of an ability to master her situation, as the next dream shows her.

Am standing on a hill that overlooks a little town. It's evening and I can see lights going on, one by one, all over town. I sit down to watch; people are walking, seem to be going home, all wearing heavy coats and knit hats. I can see their smoky breaths from the cold. However, where I'm sitting it's very warm and I have on a very lightweight cotton dress—yellow. I watch for a very long time, becoming very sleepy. I feel someone tap me on the shoulder. I turn around—it's a man, 40 or so, wearing some sort of dark green felt suit. He says, "Why are you sitting here watching?" I say, "It's so comfortable." He says, "Come on, wouldn't you rather be down there. Look, those people are dancing. Don't spend your time always watching." He touches me and suddenly he's gone. I start to cry.

It was a shock to realize that all along she had only been watching the excitement of life. Indeed she had assumed she was truly engaged in the process of living—especially since her decision to return to graduate school and to date Tom. Now she realized that even in these new contexts, she had been repeating the past and was unwilling to claim her own authority.

Confronting these current failures, Psyche took another look at her relationship with Tom. She began to see that Tom offered companionship and sexual partnership, which were quite attractive. She realized that he did not have to conform to her ideals of time spent together, or to her wishes to be protected. Remembering that she had internalized a "frantic feeling of being powerless" in her early relationships with men, she saw herself as vulnerable to the same feeling when Tom insisted on demands of his own. Finally, she contacted Tom and asked him if they could resume their relationship, a request to which he agreed after hearing about her change in attitude.

PHASE THREE: UNDERSTANDING PERSONAL RESPONSIBILITY

The final phase of therapy at this stage generally involves getting and keeping a broad perspective on one's vulnerabilities and on the human context of relationship. Acquiring a sense of what is truly personal responsibility means being able to disclaim the accidents, traumas, good luck, and fate that are not under one's control. It also means claiming the attitude of the moment as one's own and understanding how one actively constructs *self* in relation to *others* and to the events of life.

At the time of this writing, it had been more than 6 years since Psyche entered therapy. I was now seeing her for only occasional therapy sessions, most recently as she was about to take her qualifying examinations for her PhD. She was keyed up and talking rapidly. She said, "I'm afraid my all-male committee will corner me and I will feel sick to my stomach or cry." She and I reviewed the course of her development and looked realistically at her competences and coping strategies. She reminded herself that she was the author of her own work in the graduate program and that these men respected her for able, conscientious performance in their courses. Claiming for herself the idea that she deserved the good grades she had earned (especially in statistics and research design) was an important exercise, even this late in her course of therapy. No matter what level a woman's development reaches, claiming one's competences always enhances self-esteem. Psyche also credited herself with having established a vital, egalitarian relationship with Tom, whom she had recently married. She had clearly become a different woman from the one who had been so fearful and easily overwhelmed by male authority figures in the early days of her therapy.

Psyche passed her qualifying examinations and defended her dissertation proposal without succumbing to a self-deprecating or seductive manner with her professors. Her integration of the heroic animus put her in a condition of greater leadership and confidence. In the course of her treatment she had confronted, understood, and eventually integrated each of the following animus images: rapist, Father, Hephaestian demon, and Hero. As she had understood and internalized these images, assigning them a place in her personal history and in ongoing relationships, she had substantially expanded her behaviors and attitudes as a woman. Each time she had incorporated a previously rejected self-image, she felt an expanded sense of personal freedom. Paradoxically, each increase in freedom had also meant the sacrifice of a childhood attitude.

Many times during our later work, Psyche had been accompanied in dreams by an old woman figure, sometimes interpreted as a personification of me and sometimes as an aspect of herself. Psyche and I now identified this woman as a securely internalized guide figure, the archetypal Wise Old Woman, as characterized in Jung's personality theory.

In terms of the story of Amor and Psyche, I interpret this image to be like the benevolent Venus, who confers divinity on Psyche. She seems to represent an internal protection by female authority. Developmentally, she is the transformation of the old Mother complex (from childhood) into a new form of nurture and support grounded in the woman–self. As Psyche increasingly took the responsibility for her sessions in making the connecting links between behavior and symbol, the interactive field of therapy changed. Psyche and I became equal partners, true collaborators in the therapeutic process.

CONCLUDING REMARKS

Many women today are struggling to embrace the heroic animus in themselves. As this case illustrates, the embrace will always involve a confrontation with darkness and a strengthening of one's courage in honestly facing shameful and aggressive self-images. Living through the fatigue, depression, and anxiety generated by both the necessary work in the world and by the self-reflective process of development can result in liberation. An increase of peace and power, and an expanded ability to express oneself, are the products of this struggle, leading to greater respect from others and to confidence about making our own voices heard in a world which may not welcome them.

12

New Texts and Contexts for Female Development

> Unlike her male counterpart . . . the female artist must first strug-
> gle against the effects of a socialization which makes conflict with the
> will of her [male] precursors seem inexpressibly absurd, futile, or even
> . . . self-annihilating. . . . Her battle . . . is not against her [male]
> precursor's reading of the world but against his reading of *her*.
> —Gilbert and Gubar (1979, p. 49)

Our work on female authority has led us along two intertwining strands
of interpretation in psychotherapy with women. The first is a deconstruction of the animus complex, in terms of both its hidden and its
expressed convictions of male superiority. The second is a revaluation
of female socialization in terms of the myriad desires of women for their
own ideal cultural forms.

Animus deconstruction for any woman will involve reworking her
relationships with a great variety of men and boys as well as with an
omnipresent patriarchal culture that constantly makes reflections on
her intellect, power, and skills. Many levels of meaning and experience
must be pulled apart in order to understand how a woman's animus
works in her daily life. Her father may or may not be prominent in this
endeavor. The absence and distance of fathers from daughters has
resulted in women gathering their experiences of masculinity from
many sources. On the other hand, revaluation of female socialization
almost always involves a primary encounter with images of Mother.
An interpretation of the role of a client's mother and her historical life
context is often an essential element of psychotherapy.

Perhaps for this reason, most major theories of personality development share one significant error from our perspective. They confuse the *personal mother* with the *archetypal Mother complex*. This is especially true of models that psychotherapists commonly use to interpret relationships, whether psychoanalytic or systemic. Even object relations theory, with its account of "objects" as part-persons internalized from early life, depicts personality as deriving from the relationship of "the mother and her child." Reading personality from this sort of fundamental text cannot avoid burdening women with excessive feelings of responsibility for happenings of fate. To paraphrase Winnicott's famous quote "There is no such thing as a baby" (as quoted in Davis & Wallbridge, 1981, p. 34), we would say that "there is no such thing as a mother and her child." Mother and child are contained and interactive in a larger system of relationships, environment, and culture that is as important (or even more important) to personality as the female caregiver. In addition to gender, race, and social class, the family members, support systems, physical environment, material resources, and biological father (to name but a few) are major influences on personality development. Sociocultural dictates shape our complexes and are especially problematic in the contemporary Mother complex. The carrier of the Mother complex reacts to herself and to her mother through knowledge of stories told about mothers in her society.

In presenting our ideals for a new model of personality development for use (but not exclusively) with women, we emphasize the relationships between people and among complexes as these are engendered by and are expressed within society and culture. We have removed the personal mother as the cornerstone of personality. Within a configuration of competing self-images, a woman gathers an identity, which she aspires to make coherent. As we have stated elsewhere, three major motifs form the structure of our thinking about personality development in women: motivation, empathy, and meaning.

MOTIVATION: SELF AS AGENT

The experience of being one's own agent, that is, of one's own will, is a key factor in securing a personal identity and is a major concern in animus deconstruction. In fact, we believe that an adult's recognition of competence, "perceived control" (Seligman, 1975), or personal agency (MacMurray, 1957/1978) is the unifying element in being a person-among-persons, a viable member of our society. Fundamental to having a coherent identity in adulthood is the knowledge that one does things effectively, that one is useful.

Obviously this knowledge develops gradually, from infancy and reactive expressions of impulse, through childhood and learning self-control (understanding antecedents and consequences of behavior), and on to adolescence and self-reflection on will and motivations. In adulthood, personal agency is the ongoing recognition that one has a vital part to play in shaping one's own life, that one is free in making choices.

Attribution theory (e.g., Heider, 1958; Jones & Nisbett, 1971; Kelly, 1971) has contributed to psychology the premise that human motivations must be understood in terms of intentionality. Someone's discrimination between intentionality and fateful happening will be an important determinant of the meaning assigned to an event. "It makes a real difference, for example, whether a person discovers that the stick that struck him fell from a rotting tree or was hurled by an enemy" (Heider, 1958, p. 16). The attribution of intentionality to oneself or others is critical to our knowledge about the meaning of behavior. Attribution theorists have tended to focus on the distinction between impersonal happenings and personal causation.

An even more primitive (i.e., developmentally earlier) distinction is between causation by self and causation by other. The experience of "I do" in relation to "you do" comes into being in the first year of life. Notably, MacMurray (1957/1978) argues that the primacy of the personal "I do" is the conceptual basis for all theories of causation, both in science and in our experience of the physical environment.

> The "I do" . . . is the necessary starting-point. The "it happens" falls within it in actuality, and in conception is abstracted from it. I can always ask, "What happens when I do something?" when I drive a car from Glasgow to Edinburgh, for example. . . . We keep within the field of happening by excluding questions which involve a reference to agency. The moment we ask, "Why were you going to Edinburgh anyway?" the tracing of causal processes or continuant patterns must stop, because the answer must refer to an intention. (p. 160)

The idea of something happening is derived from the experience of personal agency. Human motivation is a primary factor in our understanding of causality and focal in our understanding of personality. Intentionality, of course, involves the conceptual ability to recognize one's own agency and thus to distinguish it from another's.

A woman's experience of her intentionality—and her ability to act responsibly and by free choice—is contingent upon her acceptance of personal agency. Sense of responsibility and freedom of choice are inhibited by the animus complex, however, as women exclude personal authority in their gender development. This exclusion is reinforced by social institutions that inhibit a woman's freedom and limit her equality with the opposite gender.

Theories of personality that imply that women are passive or weak (whether due to socialization or biology) and cultural institutions that limit their choice and human rights cause difficulties in establishing a personal identity in adulthood. Internalized inferiority (as animus complex) makes the logic of such theories believable to women as they become convinced of their own inherent or acquired deficits. Psychotherapeutic treatment must focus on deconstructing these beliefs in terms of both the woman's personal history and her gender identity.

In describing personal change in psychoanalysis, Schafer (1978) makes personal agency a central aim of psychoanalytic interpretation.

> . . . the analysand progressively recognizes, accepts, revises, refines, and lives in terms of the idea of the self as agent. This is to say that, in one way or another and more and more, the analysand sees himself or herself as being the person who essentially has been doing the things from which he or she was apparently suffering upon entering analysis, and from many other problems as well that will have been defined only during the analysis itself. (p. 180)

Progressive interpretation and working through of the animus complex includes understanding the ways in which a woman has contributed to her own oppression by thinking in androcentric terms. On the other hand, any client should clearly understand that she did not intend or devise her animus complex, and neither did her mother or father. Schafer offers a corollary for the aim of increasing personal agency: "Analysis also establishes progressively that it is the analysand who, unconsciously and painfully, has been arbitrarily but understandably assuming responsibility for both the fortunate and unfortunate happenings of life" (p. 180). Whether understood as fortunate or unfortunate, gender identity is clearly a happening of life. One inextricably is bound to assumptions about one's gender category until they can be deconstructed and revised.

As long as we restrict personal agency both in characteristics for "ideal women" and in social institutions in which girls grow up, we can expect serious problems in the motivational capacity of adult females. As psychotherapists, it is imperative to oppose psychological models that undermine women's beliefs in their abilities to engage actively with their own lives.

As Lipman-Blumen (1984) points out, White males dominate other groups largely through belief systems. Two prominent beliefs frequently taken as implicit assumptions are (1) that men have the necessary knowledge to master our social and cultural systems, knowledge which women do not have; and (2) that men control the major cultural resources on which women depend (p. 9). The attribution of knowledge and resources to men functions as a primary deterrent to personal motivation for change in many women we see in therapy. Rather than focus on these deficit beliefs, the therapist should assist women in delineating the knowledge and resources already under their control: that is, encourage an awareness of strength and efficacy.

Especially among women at the first two stages of animus development, experiences and descriptions of personal strengths tend to be repressed. Although full integration of personal agency may not be possible at these stages, all women can increasingly recognize the knowledge and resources under their control. Fairly reliable are some general modes of female contributions to culture and social power: emotional expressiveness, nurturance, aesthetic appearance and environments, skills in nonrational and rational communication, and empathic relating. Live art forms such as gossiping, exchanging and making recipes, keeping personal friendships, etc., will be valued more openly as we awaken our imagination to new meanings of these traditionally female activities. At the same time, of course, contributing to culture in more traditionally masculine forms is to be equally cherished—although these forms may initially be hypervalued.

Feminist theologians assist us in training our minds to spot new ideals and ideal images of female authority, and to increase our ability to see ways in which we comply with our own victimization. Daly (1978), in a radical feminist critique of androcentric religions and technology, argues that patriarchy is rooted in violent and aggressive domination of the planet and of subordinate people. She advocates a complete condemnation of patriarchal forms of power because they are inherently based on a death mode. While we are skeptical about her tendency to defensive splitting of good–bad and life–death, we are grateful for the lens she offers. Through it we become increasingly aware of the choice each of us can make in aligning our development with certain cultural forms over others, refusing to accept androcentric assumptions as truths.

Other feminist theologians, such as Ruether (1983) and Goldenberg (1979), have invited us to form ideal images of female culture and goddesses from the "shards" of buried or lost matriarchal traditions. Ruether especially emphasizes that the experiential core of feminist theology (grounded in the validity of women's perspectives on truth and goodness) needs a historical context in order to thrive. She suggests gleaning what we can from the heretical traditions (e.g., Gnosticism, Quakerism, and Shakerism) and from critical post-Christian world views (e.g, Romanticism and Marxism) in conceptualizing our ideals for the future. She cautions us about our vulnerability to dominance–submission reversals in blaming men and in projecting unwanted parts of ourselves onto the opposite gender. Her position strongly supports an ethic of equality in which human relationships are not bound by superior–inferior dualism.

Goldenberg (1979) argues, as many feminists do, that our beliefs and ideals for women must include a fundamental reconceptualization of the identity of a male god. In the Judeo-Christian tradition, the image of a male authority figure dominates every aspect of practice and faith. Consequently women are forced to exclude the validity of their own experiences and to project these onto an external locus of control. She is also critical of the classical Jungian perspective on archetypes as universal truths, asserting that this view justifies racist and sexist stereotyping and discourages cultural relativism. Opposed to a monotheistic god image, she advocates spiritual relativism in which women generate their own ideal images and stories to inspire and motivate. Since women's stories in patriarchal religions have been told by men, women must now provide their own accounts. Goldenberg emphasizes the value of psychological polytheism, derived from charting and understanding the multiple sources of one's imagination in the varying characters, motifs, and environments of dreams and fantasies.

Our aim to protect and increase personal agency in women has been clarified by reading feminist theologians who oppose religious ideals of male domination and other forms of externalizing authority. Consequently, we find ourselves often opposing common cultural dictates for success and power. For example, in evaluating her creative or work interests, a woman may automatically assume (from the perspective of animus) that the highest paid or most prestigious form of employment is best. We will urge her to examine closely the assumptions of her position. We review the potential benefits that weigh in the balance against money and status: creative expression, personal support networks, decision-making influence, integrity of values and beliefs, and needs involved with competing roles. We are not simply opposed to women using patriarchal standards of success, but we are apprehensive about assuming the validity of these categories prior to understanding how they may inhibit well-being and life satisfaction for a particular woman.

On the other hand, we have no reservations about the guidelines for personal agency that can be extrapolated from the findings of Baruch et al. (1983) regarding the importance of economic independence for women. Economic independence and work competence are core factors of personal agency for every member of our society. Challenging and imaginative work and personal sovereignty over one's finances in adult life appear critical to maintaining the experience of perceived control (Seligman, 1975) throughout one's life span. Economic independence, as an ideal, must be shaped to fit each woman's life context in therapeutic treatment. An individual woman should be considered from the "dual perspective" (Norton, 1976) of her relationship to the dominant culture and to the immediate nurturing culture of her interpersonal network. An older woman who has been financially dependent for most of her adult years, for example, will not be able to secure economic independence unless she is prepared through education or training. Even then, her age may prevent it. Consequently she must look to the material resources she has available—through social security benefits, shared rights to property and income, personal inheritance and the like—to make claims for economic independence. For some women, imaginative and useful work will be connected to economic independence and for some it will not. For all women clients, however, we encourage aspiration to ideals of material independence, and we assist them in claiming the strengths of their personal and social situations.

Younger women, especially, must be supported in their desires for education and preparation for competent work. Material self-support and creative self-interests are the two path markers we use. Multiple roles with competing responsibilities and interests (e.g., mothering and working at a paid job while going to school) are understood as healthy for women's development. As Baruch et al. (1983) report from their study of midlife American women:

> When the women in our random sample were asked about major regrets in their lives, the most common regret was abandoning their education or not pursuing career goals more seriously. The woman who manages to hang onto her career may be in for some stress in her younger years when the pulls and tugs of family and career can be intense, but if she can persist, her chances for much smoother sailing in her mature years seem very good. (p. 146)

Obviously, the dual concerns for economic independence and career competence may themselves be products of androcentric thinking and patriarchal culture. Still, they are core aspects of personal agency in our current society and must be attended as central to women's healthy identities at this time.

Imaginative ideals for female authority, ideal constructs for female contributions to culture, economic independence, freedom of choice, and cultural relativism are our guiding conceptualizations for increasing personal agency.

Since we assume that personal agency is a fundamental state of being a person-among-persons, we also use "action language" in speaking with our clients. Schafer's (1978) significant contribution to clinical method has been to specify how the language of action contributes to increasing both authority and choice in the client's perspective on her life. For example, he says:

> . . . analysands who are benefiting from analysis increasingly and appropriately present themselves as agents rather than as passive vic-

tims of happenings, be they external circumstances or seemingly autonomous inner forces and fragments of mind or a self. It becomes no longer defensively important to insist, for example, "My mind is playing tricks on me," "My anger exploded," or "Being a woman has ruined my life." (p. 186)

Even traumatic happenings are actively shaped by the individual meanings a person attributes to them. We have choices about interpretive meaning, and we are constantly constructing ourselves through such interpretation. The element of choice enters into our experience at every level when we are able to construct meaning freely. Therefore, we focus all of our interventions in an active way and oppose phrasing and ideology that victimize a person's experience of herself. Even a statement as seemingly benign as "A part of me wants to be a good mother and a part of me wants to take a long trip" can contribute to a feeling of stagnation and confusion because of the absence of personal agency in the statement. Restating her desires in personal terms such as "You want to be a good mother and you want to take a trip" clarifies her activity and choice. It also clarifies the conflict, which may have been repressed in the earlier statement.

EMPATHY: SELF AS DEPENDENT

We prefer the term "dependent" to "interdependent" because not all people are self-reliant enough to be dependable, but all people are dependent. Physical and emotional dependence is a primary condition of human life from conception until death. We assume that human dependence, as exercised and expressed in relationships, is the essential component of personality development, enacted interpersonally and symbolized intrapsychically.

Rejecting all forms of mind–body, mechanistic, object–subject, superior–inferior dualism, we embrace the concept of dependent personality. As children learn how to identify what is common to "persons" as distinct from objects and animals, they attribute personal characteristics to themselves. This learning takes place through interaction with others. We do not first discover a self and then learn to relate. There is no human process whereby certain meanings are learned privately and then noted as corresponding to others' behavior.

Learning to use and identify with all aspects of person-characteristics (i.e., person-ality) is a process of attributing them both to self and other. Thus we claim that personality is always a tandem development of self–other conceptions and never the discovery of an independent self. The fallacy of individualism, a misleading notion that we are separate units contained in private bodies like machines in little houses, leads to endless confusion about human relationship and a general repression of dependence and vulnerability. We have encountered many people—especially women—who literally believe that living alone is a condition of psychological independence. In other words, they have confused personal agency (choice, etc.) with the social condition of living alone. The idea of "living alone" is, itself, a distortion based on misconceptions about privacy because people never live alone. As organisms, we have a variety of both biological and psychological needs that prevent us from being able to survive in isolation. (Consider, for example, the prospect of being caged in a cell on a distant planet without access to nurture. Even with physical nurture in the form of food and water, the chances of remaining a person—in terms of self-reflection and personal agency—diminish considerably with the passage of time.)

The primary condition of human dependency as the basis of personality is obvious to all people who provide nurturing care for infants. Here is how MacMurray (1961) describes the adaptive nature of the human infant:

> The baby must be fitted by nature at birth to the conditions into which he [sic] is born; for otherwise he could not survive. . . . He is made to be cared for. He is born into a love-relationship which is inherently personal. Not merely his personal development, but his very survival depends upon the maintaining of this relation; he depends for his existence, that is to say, upon intelligent understanding, upon rational foresight. He cannot think for himself, yet he cannot do without thinking; so someone else must think for him. He cannot foresee his own needs. . . . It must be done for him by another who can, or he will die. (p. 48)

Thus human existence is, in principle, a shared existence. The sense of self, in its inherent structure, always refers to the other because it is the relationship to the other that provides the basis for reflection on oneself.

Our massive denial of dependence appears to be a product both of male socialization and exclusive female care in early life. Repressing their identity with (M)others of early life, men especially fight female authority and predicate their individual existence on a denial of dependence. Men then produce cultural systems which shape collective imagination around the denial of dependence and even of attachment. Men have evolved dominant models of moral and ethical reasoning based on distance and the fallacy of individualism.

In her study of moral development, Gilligan (1982) found that girls and women do not repress dependence, but continue to consider both concern and care for others to be major aspects of their development throughout childhood and adulthood.

> Thus in all of the women's descriptions, identity is defined in a context of relationship and judged by a standard of responsibility and care. Similarly, morality is seen by these women as arising from the experience of connection and conceived as a problem of inclusion rather than one of balancing claims. (p. 160)

When dependence is not repressed, a person recognizes the fundamental need for ongoing significant relationships that provide the basis for symbolic development. Within the arena of dependent relationships, we gradually distinguish "I" from "Not-I," largely on the basis of personal agency, the experience of will. Dominance–submission struggles of will between toddler and caregivers indicate that the sense of "I, me, mine" is being actualized. Around the same time, of course, gender attributes become significant. Adult caretakers label actions as "little girl" or "little boy" and begin to shape the activities of the two genders into the roles in which they will serve the society.

The way we see it, girls emerge into the larger social world quite consciously connected to dependency needs and to their identification with (M)other of early life. Boys, on the other hand, are forced to deny and repress both the felt dependency needs and the identification with (M)other, creating a more primitive and split-off Mother complex. Through school and adolescence the gap between girls and boys widens in this regard. Girls are encouraged to perceive and feel dependence and vulnerability. Boys are encouraged to see themselves as independent of emotional needs, and of their own weaknesses or vulnerabilities. Concomitantly, boys must see themselves in competitive opposition to other boys, as rationally distant from other personalities, and as motivationally distinct from girls and women and their interests.

In same-sex peer relationships of childhood and adolescence, girls have greater access to mutual sharing and emotional intimacy with each other. According to Sullivan (1953), it is just this type of "chum" relationship that provides the basis later for responsibility, reciprocity, and authentic moral conscience. True equality and altruism are rooted in peer relationships, according to Sullivan, and not in dominant–submission relationships with parents (although certain rules may be set in the latter). Not until a person has experienced a dependent relationship with an equal whom one values as much as (not more or less) than oneself, can a person understand the merit of being responsible for one's actions, desires, and feelings as these affect another.

Most girls and women approach intimate male–female relationships in adolescence and adulthood expecting mutual trust and sharing. Due to the animus complex, they also anticipate validation and approval.

The combination of desire for trusting dependence and desire for validation makes a girl vulnerable to the kind of "identity relationship" we have described in detail. This projection of her most cherished ideals onto the male is different from "identity *in* relationship," which is a central ideal of our model of personality development.

The struggle that ensues from a woman's desire for trusting dependence in adulthood generally results in her assuming that her desire is inferior and perhaps even in denigrating her own needs. This struggle, of course, combines with enactments and identifications with the negative Mother complex and tends to increase the anxiety arising from animus.

As we have said elsewhere, it is our aim to strengthen and validate a woman's needs for emotional dependence while differentiating these from material dependence and personal agency.

Our ultimate aim is to increase objective empathy in our clients as we support their desires for relationship and their ability to perceive both intended and unintended meanings in human communications. Because they are aware of their dependency needs, many women have "feminine intuition." That is, they can accurately read communications from others on a variety of levels, especially regarding emotional meanings. Truly objective empathy, as stated elsewhere, is a mature developmental achievement, which evolves from symbiosis, projection, and sympathy, but is distinct from these. A term from ordinary language comes close to what we mean by objective empathy: *compassion*. Compassion is accurate awareness of another's distress with a desire to relieve it.

We find that increasing female authority often leads to increased empathy and compassion as a woman acknowledges her strengths in her ability to relate to others. In order to do this, however, she must be secure in her personal agency and aware of her motivational independence. Our experiences in working with women to retrieve authority and deconstruct animus assumptions certainly support Gilligan's (1982) observations that

> . . . women's sense of integrity appears to be entwined with an ethic of care, so that to see themselves as women is to see themselves in a relationship of connection. . . . When the distinction between helping and pleasing frees the activity of taking care from the wish for approval by others, the ethic of responsibility can become a self-chosen anchor of personal integrity and strength. (p. 171)

Two general therapeutic goals provide a basis for increasing empathy and compassion in human relationship. The first has already been discussed in detail: repeatedly supporting and validating needs for emotional dependence. The second specifically involves the component of "objectivity" in empathic regard. As was mentioned in Chapter 4, women sometimes have difficulty reinstating a sense of self and communicating observations of empathic regard. This is generally a problem with the negative Mother complex through which they have berated themselves for feeling dependent and vulnerable, for being "irrational," or whatever. We encourage women to find their own words and to express confidently their intuitive observations. They learn to sort out the anxieties of their self-denigrations from the emotional expressions of other people. When they can do this accurately and regularly, they can develop a rational language for empathic expression, which is a valuable tool in forming a dialectical relationship both with others and with themselves.

The ideal of objective empathy for another or for oneself is not based on a subject–object dichotomy of observer and observed. Rather it is an articulation of the idea that we can know what is common or universal in personal experience from self–other reflections. MacMurray (1961) captures this idea in the following passage:

> This original reference to the other is of a definitive importance. It is the germ of rationality. For the character that distinguishes rational from non-rational experience, in all the expressions of reason, is its reference to the Other-than-myself. What we call "objectivity" is one expression of this—the conscious reference of an idea to an object. But it is to be noted that this is not the primary expression of reason. What is primary, even in respect of reflective thought—is the reference to the other *person*. . . . Objective thought presupposes this by the assumption that there is a *common* object about which a communication may be made. (p. 61, italics in original)

MacMurray's point here agrees with our own observations. In true empathic regard there is a blending of the highest subjectivity and the highest objectivity. That is, through the woman's personal experience of the other—whether it is a dependent child or an equal partner—she can intuit or perceive much that is accurate about the "private" or emotional state of being of the other. Our cultural mistrust of this kind of perception can lead us, as psychotherapists, to confuse empathy with fusion and projection.

Both the initial impulse for symbolic activity and the ongoing reality of symbolic communication seem to arise out of the mutuality of human existence. Out of the primitive dialogue of "you and I" comes a dynamic that eventually constitutes self-reflection and person-ality.

MEANING: SELF AS ARTIST

Many times in our work, we have referred to the metaphor of spinning or weaving for the process of constructing a female self from competing desires and conflicting complexes. We believe that this metaphor is a good one for the kind of activity in which we are involved: unraveling the knots of animus introjections and mending the fragmented consciousness of female culture. To believe in ourselves as artists who can create a new tapestry of meaning from our repressed desires and "unweave the ghostly false images of ourselves which have been deeply embedded in our imaginations" (Daly, 1978, p. 409) is to engender female authority.

Reconstruction of meaning through psychotherapy generally involves directing our attention to conflicts between nonrational or unintended meanings and rational or intended meanings. Nonrational modes of communication include gestural expressions, projected attitudes and desires, dreams, transference of parental and animus complexes onto others, and other distorted irrational thoughts about oneself or another. The therapeutic relationship is itself arranged to emphasize the incongruent or conflicting aspects of collaboration with a knowledgeable expert. An effective therapeutic relationship instigates a paradoxical opposition between cooperation and resistance. Although the client comes with the intention of revealing what has been distressing her, and/or with the purpose of getting some kind of help, she soon discovers that she resists or fails to understand the therapist's meaning at a crucial juncture. It is this failure that opens the door to change.

This paradoxical aspect of the therapeutic relationship distinguishes it from other forms of helpful relationships, such as with family members and friends. By ritual and arrangement, therapy emphasizes the conflicted aspects of symbolic communication and personal contract so that unintended desires naturally arise with regard to such concerns as love, money, time, aggression, and appearances.

In order to weave a new fabric of personal meaning, a woman must undo her animus rationalizations around her conviction of inferiority. We find that this is the tough core of resistance and often the most inflexible aspect of her personality, especially when a woman is in the first two stages of animus development. While vulnerable to defensively splitting negative animus qualities and to blaming herself and the men around her for her condition, a woman may seem rigid in her belief that she is unworthy of healing and love. Working through alien and father–god animus complexes is the most difficult work we do in unweaving false images. We are reminded of the statement made by Jung (1966) about his therapeutic aim: "My aim is to bring about a psychic state in which my patient begins to experiment with his [sic] own nature—a state of fluidity, change, and growth where nothing is eternally fixed, and hopelessly petrified" (p. 46). The most "hopelessly petrified" and "eternally fixed" meanings arise from Stage One and Stage Two animus complexes. Working through the complex (in analysis or a corrective emotional relationship) reveals to a client the way in which she has attempted to purge herself of her aggressive impulses, her own truths, and her personal worth.

Although much could be said about the metaphor of weaving new meanings from the fragments of female identity, we have chosen one motif that arises in almost every treatment as a prototype of meaning recontruction. Originating in a Pandora adaptation, and crucial to an authentic self at all later stages, is the conflict of beauty and the "beast," that is, appearance as power.

In our discussion of the Pandora stage (Chaps. 6, 9, and 10) we have stressed the aspect of approval as the motivating force in a woman's desire to "look good" and "make nice." Approval seeking is the culturally condoned mode by which a woman may identify herself with the powerful other onto whom she has projected her own authority. At this stage, a woman strives to be conventionally pretty or successful through "looking good" from the male perspective. Her relationship to her Pandora facade usually has some individual aesthetic in it, but it is designed to meet the standards of the external authorities over and above her own desires.

At later stages of development, we distinguish a woman's desire for beauty in herself and her environment from mere approval seeking. As Brownmiller (1984) points out, women's appearances—through skin, hair, clothes, etiquette, and body shape—convey essential social meanings. Stereotyped perceptions and expectations concerning appearances often result in comments that imply a woman *is* her appearance. An unkempt or plump woman may hear that she "has let *herself* go." This wholly undifferentiated way of thinking about women's appearances is a problem for women at later stages of development, both in their self-assessments and in their interpersonal associations, especially with other women. As a culture, we seem caught at the Pandora stage (or alternatively at Loevinger's Self-Protective and Conformist Stages) when it comes to evaluating woman as appearance.

Women who have developed beyond the Pandora orientation (having differentiated own desires from animus complex) are propelled into an existential conflict about what we might call "appearance and reality." At the Psyche stage, for example, a woman may disavow her earlier acceptance of a formula for beautiful appearance (i.e., appearance = self-worth), but not be able to reestablish her relatedness to the idea of her beauty. She will tend to be polarized in her thinking about appearance: She does not want to identify herself with traditional femininity or artifice, but she continues to be aware of the social power afforded her if she does. Consequently, she may rebel through her appearance itself ("letting herself go") and not control her weight, not shave her legs, wear makeup, etc. In this way she implies that she refuses to equate artifice and reality; she refuses to distort herself by assuming a facade. Similarly, she may rebel against masculine forms of success, and abandon traditional education, employment, etc., in the patriarchy.

In her rebellious freedom (which, of course, is still bound to the cultural dictates of acceptable appearance for women), she discovers new comforts. She observes, "I really don't like wearing high-heeled shoes and nylon stockings." Because she has not yet clearly differentiated her animus assumptions about these, she believes that her truth belongs to other women as well. She will tend to categorize women by their appearance and assume that if they are groomed in feminine ways they are conformist "antifeminist," or unevolved. Thus she is engaged in the very trap she sought to escape by becoming more expressive of her "real self" in opposing the conventional dictates about women's appearances. This polarization of self-worth and appearance is depicted in the struggle of Psyche at the end of the Amor and Psyche tale. She is exhausted from the travails of her own seeking and decides that she will claim some of the beauty in Persephone's box for herself (it rightly belongs to Venus, with whom she has a contract). When Psyche opens the box she is overwhelmed by its contents and sinks into apparent death. Venus, the goddess of Beauty and Love, restores Psyche to her powerful divinity at the end of the story.

What happens here psychologically? From our clinical work and from our own lives, we believe that women eventually come to understand and embrace both beauty and artifice as female cultural resources (aspects of their socialization) when they integrate animus. Beauty—connected to personal integrity—is rightfully a part of an integrated lifestyle. Artifice, connected to personal power and influence, is also rightfully part of a woman's resources. When women, those at the last two stages, come to recognize the personal meaning of beauty and artifice, and to differentiate them consciously and understand their cultural meanings, they can use them discriminately with integrity. Until this takes place, most woman are vulnerable to depression and loss of self-worth in regard to their appearance because of the social conditions under which we live.

We include ideals for beautiful appearance and creative use of beauty in the environment within our aims for animus development. Our concerns over this issue, from the point of view of ideal development, rest especially in problems we have observed in women who hurt each other by competing for beauty and by denigrating the beauty of others. At the Psyche stage especially, responsible young women and otherwise sensitive older women may depreciate their peers for adherence to feminine or androgynous cultural styles.

In general, we encourage our clients toward a more differentiated use of appearance and receptivity to other women's appearances. The defensive attitude of a Pandora orientation to appearances is recognized by the splitting or polarization of women's appearances into categories of feminine–masculine, pretty–ugly, bright–dumb, etc. This attitude is often used in regressive moments of lowered self-esteem beyond the Pandora stage itself. Deconstructing animus assumptions about women's appearances and reality is an ongoing project of consciousness raising in a society that gives double-binding messages about feminine power as appearance.

The metaphor of woman as artist can be used to unravel many aspects of our assumed identities. Appearance is an especially rich and conflicted topic regarding female psychology. We use it to illustrate the process by which old meanings are pulled apart and new ones are constructed through psychotherapy. In meaning reconstruction, one of our most serious aims is the rebonding of women and the integration of the female community. Competition and deficit labeling among women are animus-related activities in general. As we pull apart the assumptions that lead us to denigrate each other we increasingly find that the projection of authority (the externalization of control) is the central most devisive factor in women's relationships to each other. As quoted earlier regarding the ethic of care, Gilligan (1982) said, "When the distinction between helping and pleasing frees the activity of taking care from the wish for approval by others, the ethic of responsibility can become a self-chosen anchor of personal integrity and strength" (p. 171). The same distinction between beauty and pleasing frees the activity of self-expression to be anchored in personal integrity and strength.

> She is the one you call sister.
> Her simplest act has glamor,
> as when she scales a fish the knife
> flashes in her long fingers
> no motion wasted. . . .
> (Rich, 1984b)

CONCLUDING REMARKS

We have set out ideals for a new model of personality development with the full knowledge that we are working on a project that is shared with many others under social conditions which are often unsupportive. It is our hope that the collective enthusiasm and the imagination needed for a new understanding of human personality will pull us through this difficult period of human culture, as we all become more acutely aware of the dangers of annihilation that face our species. Firm recognition of our dependence on each other, the interpersonal nature of personality, and the meaning of human freedom (as personal agency) may assist us in acquiring the kind of objective empathy we need to survive.

If not, our species may go the way of many other life forms whose adaptation eventually led to extinction. As relatively weak animals, we have acquired an enormous dominion of power through our inherent impulses for narcissistic control. We have seemed unable to imagine a world in which the human being is not in control—a world of natural resources, of other human beings, even of fate itself.

On the other hand, we are also certainly aware that we are not in control of our own destiny. Our fate is individual extinction and a life on a small planet dependent on a relatively small star in a solar system which will inevitably dissolve. The psychological conflict of control and dependency is unique to human life, but we must imagine ourselves as compassionate beings in order to make our shared existence meaningful. As women, we believe that this is a critical time for contributing our female authority, our knowledge that dependence is the absolute boundary of personality.

REFERENCES

Albee, G., & Joffe, J. (Eds.). (1977). *Primary prevention of psychopathology: The issues* (Vol. 1). Hanover, NH: University Press of New England.

American Psychiatric Association. (1980). *Diagnostic and statistical manual of mental disorders* (3rd ed.). Washington, DC: Author.

Bardwick, J. M., Douvan, E., Horner, M. S., & Gutmann, D. (1970). *Feminine personality and conflict*. Westport, CT: Greenwood Press.

Barry, H., Bacon, M. K., & Child, I. L. (1957). A cross-cultural survey of some sex differences in socialization. *Journal of Abnormal and Social Psychology, 55*, 327–332.

Baruch, G., Barnett, R., & Rivers, C. (1983). *Life prints: New patterns of love and work for today's woman*. New York: McGraw-Hill, 1983.

Bem, S. L., Martyna, W., & Watson, C. (1976). Sex typing and androgyny: Further explorations of the expressive domain. *Journal of Personality and Social Psychology, 34*, 1016–1023.

Benedek, T. F. (1952). Infertility as a psychosomatic defense. *Fertility and Sterility, 3*, 527–541.

Benedek, T. F. (1959). Sexual functions in women and their disturbance. In S. Arieti (Ed.), *American handbook of psychiatry* (p. 726). New York: Basic Books.

Bernard, J. (1972). *The future of marriage*. New York: World.

Block, J. H. (1973). Conceptions of sex role: Some cross cultural and longitudinal perspectives. *American Psychologist, 28*, 512–526.

Bond, L., & Rosen, J. (Eds.). (1980). *Competence and coping during adulthood*. Hanover, NH: University Press of New England.

Bowlby, J. (1969). *Attachment and loss* (Vol. 1). London: Hogarth Press.

Brannigan, G., & Tolor, A. (1971). Sex differences in adaptive styles. *Journal of Genetic Psychology, 119*, 143–149.

Brodsky, A. M., & Hare-Mustin, R. T. (Eds.). (1980). *Women and psychotherapy: An assessment of research and practice*. New York: Guilford Press.

Broverman, I. K., Broverman, D. M., Clarkson, F. E., Rosenkrantz, P. S., & Vogel, S. R. (1970). Sex-role stereotypes and clinical judgements of mental health. *Journal of Consulting and Clinical Psychology, 34*, 1–7.

Broverman, I. K., Vogel, S. R., Broverman, D. M., Clarkson, F. E., & Rosenkrantz, P. S. (1972). Sex-role stereotypes: A current appraisal. *Journal of Social Issues, 28*, 59–78.

Brownmiller, S. (1984). *Femininity*. New York: Ballantine.

Chernin, K. (1981). *The obsession: Reflections on the tyranny of slenderness*. New York: Harper & Row.

Chertok, L., Mondzain, M. L., & Bonnaud, M. (1963). Vomiting and the wish to have a child. *Psychosomatic Medicine, 25*, 13–18.

Chodorow, N. (1978). *The reproduction of mothering: Psychoanalysis and the sociology of gender*. Berkeley, CA: University of California Press.

Claremont de Castillejo, I. (1973). *Knowing woman: A feminine psychology*. New York: Harper & Row.

Dally, A. (1982). *Inventing motherhood: The consequences of an ideal*. New York: Schocken Books.

Dalton, K. (1964). *The premenstrual syndrome*. Springfield, IL: Charles C. Thomas.

Daly, M. (1978). *Gyn/ecology: The metaethics of radical feminism*. Boston: Beacon Press.

Dan, A. J. (1976). *Behavioral variability and the menstrual cycle*. Paper presented at the 84th Annual Convention of the American Psychological Association, Washington, DC.

Davis, M., & Wallbridge, D. (1981). *Boundary and space: An introduction to the work of D. W. Winnicott*. New York: Brunner/Mazel.

Deutsch, H. (1944). *The psychology of women: A psychoanalytic interpretation* (Vol. 1). New York: Grune & Stratton.

Deutsch, H. (1945). *The psychology of women: A psychoanalytic interpretation* (Vol. 2). New York: Grune & Stratton.

Devereux, G. (1960). The female castration complex and its repercussions in modesty, appearance, and courtship etiquette. *American Images, 17*, 3–19.

Dinnerstein, D. (1976). *The mermaid and the minotaur: Sexual arrangements and human malaise*. New York: Harper & Row.

Douvan, E. (1970). New sources of conflict in females at adolescence and early adulthood. In J. M. Bardwick, E. Douvan, M. S. Horner, & D. Gutmann (Eds.), *Feminine personality and conflict* (pp. 31–43). Westport, CT: Greenwood Press.

Dowling, C. (1981). *The cinderella complex: Woman's hidden fear of independence*. New York: Simon & Schuster.

Eagly, A. (1983). Gender and social influence: A social psychological analysis. *American Psychologist, 38*, 971–981.

Ehrenreich, B. (1983). *The hearts of men: American dreams and the flight from commitment*. Garden City, NY: Anchor Press/Doubleday.

Erikson, E. H. (1968). *Identity: Youth and crisis*. New York: Norton.

Freud, S. (1953). Fragment of an analysis of a case of hysteria. In J. Strachey (Ed. and Trans.), *The standard edition of the complete psychological works of Sigmund Freud* (Vol. 7, pp. 7–122). London: Hogarth Press. (Original work published 1905.)

Gilbert, S. M., & Gubar, S. (1979). *The madwoman in the attic: The woman writer and the nineteenth-century literary imagination*. New Haven, CT: Yale University Press.

Gilligan, C. (1982). *In a different voice: Psychological theory and women's development*. Cambridge, MA: Harvard University Press.

Goldenberg, N. (1979). *Changing the gods: Femininism and the end of traditional religions.* Boston: Beacon Press.

Goldfarb, W., Goldfarb, N., & Scholl, H. (1966). The speech of mothers of schizophrenic children. *American Journal of Psychiatry, 122,* 1220–1227.

Gove, W. R. (1972). The relationship between sex roles, marital status and mental illness. *Social Forces, 51,* 34–44.

Grant, M. (1962). *Myths of the Greeks and Romans.* New York: New American Library/Mentor.

Hare-Mustin, R. T. (1983). An appraisal of the relationship between women and psychotherapy: 80 years after the case of Dora. *American Psychologist, 38,* 593–601.

Harvey, W. A., & Sherfey, M. J. (1954). Vomiting in pregnancy: A psychiatric study. *Psychosomatic Medicine, 16,* 1–9.

Heider, F. (1958). *The psychology of interpersonal relations.* New York: Wiley.

Heilbrun, A. B. (1968). Sex roles: Instrumental–expressive behavior, and psychopathology in females. *Journal of Abnormal Psychology, 73,* 131–136.

Holt, R. (1980). Loevinger's measure of ego development: Reliability and national norms for male and female short forms. *Journal of Personality and Social Psychology, 39,* 909–920.

Horney, K. (1933). Maternal conflicts. In H. Kelman (Ed.), *Feminine psychology* (pp. 175–181). New York: Norton.

Ivey, M. E., & Bardwick, J. M. (1968). Patterns of affective fluctuation in the menstrual cycle. *Psychosomatic Medicine, 30*(3), 336–345.

Jones, E. E., & Nisbett, R. E. (1971). The actor and the observer: Divergent perceptions of the causes of behavior. In E. E. Jones, D. E. Kanouse, H. H. Kelly, R. E. Nisbett, S. Valins, & B. Weiner (Eds.), *Attribution: Perceiving the causes of behavior* (pp. 79–94). Morristown, NJ: General Learning Press.

Jordan, J. V. (1983). Empathy and the mother–daughter relationship. *Work in Progress, 2,* 2–5.

Jung, C. G. (1959). *The collected works of C. G. Jung: Aion* (2nd ed., Vol. 9, Part II) (R. F. C. Hull, Trans.). Princeton, NJ: Princeton University Press.

Jung, C. G. (1966). *The collected works of C. G. Jung: The practice of psychotherapy* (Vol. 16) (R. F. C. Hull, Trans.). Princeton, NJ: Princeton University Press.

Jung, C. G. (1969a). *The collected works of C. G. Jung: The archetypes and the collective unconscious* (2nd ed., Vol. 9, Part I) (R. F. C. Hull, Trans.). Princeton, NJ: Princeton University Press.

Jung, C. G. (1969b). *The collected works of C. G. Jung: The structure and dynamics of the psyche* (2nd ed., Vol. 8) (R. F. C. Hull, Trans.). Princeton, NJ: Princeton University Press.

Kelly, H. H. (1971). Causal schemata and the attribution process. In E. E. Jones, D. E. Kanouse, H. H. Kelly, R. E. Nisbett, S. Valins, & B. Weiner (Eds.), *Attribution: Perceiving the causes of behavior* (pp. 151–174). Morristown, NJ: General Learning Press.

Kerenyi, C. (1974). *The gods of the Greeks.* London: Thames & Hudson.

Klein, M. (1932). *The psycho-analysis of children* (A. Strachey, Trans.). London: Hogarth Press.

Kohlberg, L. (1981). *The philosophy of moral development*. San Francisco: Harper & Row.

Kravetz, D., & Jones, L. (1981). Androgyny as a standard of mental health. *American Journal of Orthypsychiatry, 51*, 502–509.

Langs, L., & Searles, H. F. (1980). *Intrapsychic and interpersonal dimensions of treatment*. New York: Jason Aronson.

Levitt, E. E., & Lubin, B. (1967). Some personality factors associated with menstrual complaints and menstrual attitudes. *Journal of Psychosomatic Research, 11*, 267–270.

Lipman-Blumen, J. (1984). *Gender roles and power*. Englewood Cliffs, NJ: Prentice-Hall.

Loevinger, J. (1976). *Ego development*. San Francisco: Jossey-Bass.

Loevinger, J., & Wessler, R. (1970). *Measuring ego development I: Construction and use of a sentence completion test*. San Francisco: Jossey-Bass.

Loewald, H. W. (1951). Ego and reality. *International Journal of Psycho-Analysis, 32*, 10–18.

Maccoby, E. E., & Jacklin, C. N. (1974). *The psychology of sex differences* (Vol. 1). Stanford, CA: Stanford University Press.

MacMurray, J. (1961). *Persons in relation*. Atlantic Highlands, NJ: Humanities Press.

MacMurray, J. (1978). *The self as agent*. Atlantic Highlands, NJ: Humanities Press. (Original work published 1957.)

Mahler, M., Pine, F., & Bergman, A. (1975). *The psychological birth of the infant: Symbiosis and individuation*. New York: Basic Books.

Miller, J. B. (1976). *Toward a new psychology of women*. Boston: Beacon Press.

Money, J. (1976). Differentiation of gender identity. *JSAS Catalog of Selected Documents in Psychology, 6*(4).

Money, J., & Ehrhardt, A. A. (1972). *Man and woman, boy and girl: The differentiation and dimorphism of gender identity from conception to maturity*. Baltimore, MD: Johns Hopkins University Press.

Neumann, E. (1959). The psychological stages of feminine development. *Spring*, 63–97.

Norton, D. (1976). Working with minority populations: The dual perspective. In B. Ross & S. Khinduka (Eds.), *Social work in practice* (pp. 134–141). Washington, DC: National Association of Social Workers.

Parlee, M. B. (1973). The premenstrual syndrome. *Psychological Bulletin, 80*, 454–465.

Piaget, J. (1926). *The language and thought of the child* (M. Warden, Trans.). New York: Harcourt, Brace.

Rich, A. (1976). *Of woman born*. New York: Norton.

Rich, A. (1984a). Diving into the wreck. In *The fact of a doorframe, Poems selected and new, 1950–1984*. New York: Norton.

Rich, A. (1984b). The mirror in which two are seen as one. In *The fact of a doorframe, Poems selected and new, 1950–1984*. New York: Norton.

Rotter, J. B. (1966). Generalized expectancies for internal versus external control of reinforcements. *Psychological Monographs, 80*(609) (Special issue).

Ruether, R. (1983). *Sexism and god-talk*. Boston: Beacon Press.

Schafer, R. (1978). *Language and insight*. New Haven, CT: Yale University Press.

Schafer, R. (1983). *The analytic attitude*. New York: Basic Books.

Searles, H. F. (1965). *Collected papers on schizophrenia and related subjects*. New York: International Universities Press.

Sears, R. R. (1970). Relation of early socialization experiences to self-concepts and gender role in middle childhood. *Child Development, 41,* 267–289.

Seligman, M. E. P. (1975). *Helplessness: On depression, development, and death*. San Francisco: Freeman.

Shereshefsky, P. M. (1970). The childbearing experience: Is anatomy destiny? *Child and Family, 9,* 4–33.

Sherif, C. W. (1982). Needed concepts in the study of gender identity. *Psychology of Women Quarterly, 6,* 378–388.

Stevens, A. (1982). *Archetypes: A natural history of the self*. New York: Morrow.

Stiver, I. (1983). Work inhibitions in women: Clinical considerations. *Stone Center Work in Progress Papers, 82,* 1–11.

Sullivan, H. S. (1953). *The interpersonal theory of psychiatry*. New York: Norton.

Thurnher, M. (1983). Turning points and developmental change: Subjective and "objective" assessments. *American Journal of Orthopsychiatry, 53,* 52–60.

Ullian, D. Z. (1981). Why boys will be boys: A structural perspective. *American Journal of Orthopsychiatry, 51,* 493–501.

Whiting, B., & Whiting, J. (1975). *Children of six cultures: A psycho-cultural analysis*. Cambridge, MA: Harvard University Press.

Williams, J. H. (1974). *Psychology of women: Behavior in a biosocial context*. New York: Norton.

Woodman, M. (1982). *Addiction to perfection: The still unravished bride*. Toronto, Canada: Inner City Books.

Wooley, S. C., & Wooley, O. W. (1980). Eating disorders: Obesity and anorexia. In A. M. Brodsky & R. T. Hare-Mustin (Eds.), *Women and psychotherapy: An assessment of research and practice* (pp. 135–158). New York: Guilford Press.

Young-Eisendrath, P. (1984). *Hags and heroes: A feminist approach to Jungian psychotherapy with couples*. Toronto: Inner City Books.

INDEX

Anxiety and motherhood, 149
Aphrodite. *See* Venus (Aphrodite)
Appearance, 229, 230
Apuleius, 115
Archetype, 36–39, 42
Ariadne and Theseus, 144–147, 154, 156
Attribution theory, 217
Authority, female, 8–11
  compared with ego autonomy, 10, 11
  and development, 53
  male fight against, 223
  therapeutic help, 65–68
Authority, restoration of, 139–157
  aggression/rage, 143, 144
  animus development, 155–157
    as Androgyne, 153–155; as Partner
    Within, 139, 143, 144
  Ariadne and Theseus, 144–147, 154, 156
  case histories
    Alma, 151, 152; Andrea, 154; Diane,
    149, 150
  fears of abandonment, 142–147
  motherhood, 139, 140, 149–151
  objective empathy, 148, 150, 154, 155
  overaccommodation, 141
  prestige job and children, 141, 142
  therapeutic strategies, 147–153
  trusting men, 152, 153
Autonomous Stage, 64–65, 136

Baruch, G., 113, 141, 142, 221
Beauty and achievement confused, 90, 92
Betrayal fantasies, 172–174, 176, 193
Bull/minotaur, 144, 146

Career
  versus family, 30, 141, 142
  job dissatisfaction, 161, 166–168, 176,
    177, 187, 190, 191, 195, 196
  move out of graduate school to job,
    160, 161, 166
Case histories
  Alma, 151, 152
  Andrea, 132–134, 154
  Annette, 69–71
  April, 107–109
  Connie, 127, 128
  Diane, 136, 137, 149, 150
  Dora (Freud), 94, 95
  Leah, 85
  Linda, 121, 122, 129, 135, 136
  Lucy, 96, 97
  Maddy, 97–99
  Maude, 86, 87, 125, 126, 131, 132
  Patty, 103, 104, 109, 110
  Wanda, 107
Case histories, Pandora, 158–201
  analysis of case, 196–198
  assessment, 162–164

betrayal fantasies, 172–174, 176, 193
boyfriend Dan, loss, 160, 161, 166,
  168, 170, 174, 195
crying, 176, 177, 185
domineering Father, 163, 167–169, 182,
  189–191
dreams, 176, 178, 191, 192
  Bob's infidelity, 199; breast lump,
  male doctor, 167; dead person in
  apartment, 193; father in hospital,
  183–185; father's murder, 178–182,
  191; hostage, seduction, 166; Jackson, Michael, 200; jewelry in street,
  199; Jungian seminar, kiss, 165; man
  at office party, 168; mother in
  asylum, 201; negative animus complex (Black man), 181–185, 192, 198–
  200; piano, masturbation, 168, 169;
  president of corporation, 195; rescue
  from Blacks by Bob, 198; sister's
  wedding, 171; skating on thin ice,
  166; spray can in bed with Bob, 170;
  swampy Father complex, 174;
  woman's apartment, massage, 173
financial concerns, 189–191
Hephaestus, 173, 178, 190, 195
identity relationship, 169–175, 177,
  178, 183, 187, 191–201
job dissatisfaction, 161, 166, 167, 176,
  177, 187, 190, 191, 195, 196
monsters within, cute, 185, 186
mother in shell, 162, 163, 168, 196, 197
move out of graduate school to job,
  160, 161, 166
negative Mother complex, 189–191,
  197, 200, 201
parents' sexual encounters, 194
persona development, 175, 177
Self-Aware Stage, 164
separation from parents, 170–174, 182
sister Emma, 179, 180
therapeutic goals, 164, 165
therapist as father, 165
transcript of session, 176–193
worthlessness, feelings of, 178, 192
Case histories, Psyche, 202–214
  abuse, sexual, 204–208, 210
  dental hygienist, 203, 206
  difficulty conceiving, 203
  divorce as death marriage, 203
  dreams
    in bed with professor, 211, 212;
    clothes in locked cabinet, 211; hit-
    ting mother with broom, 206; mir-
    ror, alfalfa sprouts on head, 205;
    with mother in car, 207; old wom-
    an, 214; psychology class, 209, 210;
    rock fusing together, 209, 210; statue,
    demon, in boat, 207, 208; watching